Safeguard Your Ambulatory Nursing Care
Practice: How To Avoid Legal Risks

Patricia Iyer MSN RN LNCC

Pat Iyer Group
Fort Myers, FL

Safeguard Your Ambulatory Care Nursing Practice: How To Avoid Legal Risks

This product is for sale. Purchase a copy at www.legalnursebusiness.com.

Cover design and layout by Jessica Wilson

Published by:
The Pat Iyer Group
11205 Sparkleberry Drive,
Fort Myers, FL 33913
908-391-7933
www.legalnursebusiness.com

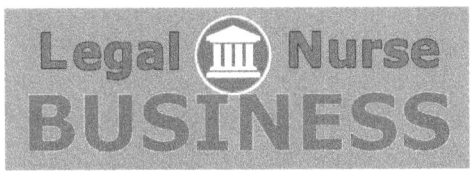

About the Author

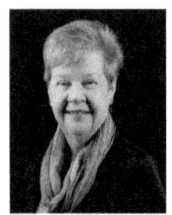

PATRICIA W. IYER, MSN RN LNCC

President

The Pat Iyer Group – education for legal nurse consultants
www.legalnursebusiness.com

Fort Myers, FL

Patricia Iyer is president of The Pat Iyer Group. She assists
legal nurse consultants to skyrocket their businesses. Her
coaching academy, LNCAcademyinc.com, provides
education, support, encouragement and networking
opportunities. She has been a legal nurse consultant since
1987 when she first began reviewing cases as an expert
witness. She achieved national prominence through her
texts and many contributions to the legal nurse consulting
field. She was the chief editor of *Legal Nurse Consulting
Principles and Practices, Second Edition*, the core curriculum for
legal nurse consulting. She completed 5 years on the Board of
Directors of the American Association of Legal Nurse
Consulting including a term as president.

Reach Pat at patriciaiyer@gmail.com

"I have been a legal nurse consultant colleague of Pat Iyer's for almost 10 years. She is considered a leader among legal nurse consultants and has written multiple books on this subject which have offered guidance to us all. She is highly respected in her profession."
—*Kathy G. Ferrell, BS, RN, LNCC*

"Pat is an exceptional person who is highly dedicated and creative. She has excelled in many areas of health care and pioneered many aspects. It is a pleasure to be affiliated with Pat."
—*Kathy Martin, Legal Nurse Consultant*

"Patricia is on one of the founders of legal nurse consulting. She has contributed substantially to the profession's growth as a leader in the field. I would highly recommend Patricia in this field."
—*Jane Barone, Legal Nurse Consultant and Author*

"I worked with Patricia on a book project as one of her contributors and she was incredible. Professional and easy to work with — I don't know what else a person could ask for."
—*Diane Wiley, Legal Nurse Consultant and Author*

" . . . Great information and very comprehensive. If you need more information, please look at Pat Iyer's website and buy some of her programs. They will be well worth your money.
—*Kathie Condon, Legal Nurse Consultant*

"I want to tell you about a wonderful website I found online: Avoid Medical Errors. If you become a member of the Inner Circle, you can gain valuable information for yourself and your family member. This website actually provides you with the information you need so you can prevent any medical errors occurring with your loved ones."
—*Lynn Fauerbach, RN*

"Pat is prolific author, extremely good. I have a shelf in my study, bookcase area that is just hers. I learned a lot from her."
—*Pat Bemis, Past President of National Nurses in Business*

Pat's legal presentation at the Academy of medical Surgical Nursing was thoughtful. It was engaging. It was interesting. It was well-thought out. I came away from that presentation with a lot of information I can take back to the staff where I work. We can tweak our practice and we can document in a more thoughtful manner. I would always go to a presentation that Pat was a part of.
—*Linda Willette, RN*

I have had the pleasure and honor of meeting Pat Iyer. She is so professional. Just watching her has inspired me as a family nurse practitioner to be more professional. She has given workshops and speaking engagements. Everyone has attested to her knowledge in the field. She has written books. I wish that you too could take the opportunity to meet with her. She has a website. Take advantage of some of the materials she has to offer.
—*Leslie Lee RN MSN*

Preface

You have a special opportunity to provide nursing care in the ambulatory care setting. The roles and practice settings of ambulatory care nurses are unique. You have the honor of educating and assessing patients and making a difference in the lives of those you serve.

The complexities of health care make patient injury a reality; we all need to do our best to minimize the risk of injury. There are few events more disturbing to nurses than to find out they are being sued for nursing malpractice. The first reaction may be bewilderment, followed by anger. The intent of this book is to help you understand your risks as an ambulatory care nurse so you can take proactive action to reduce the risk of patient harm and lawsuits. This book will take you by the hand and lead you through the legal process. You'll learn concrete strategies you can put into action to protect your patients as well as yourself.

You will benefit from my extensive knowledge as a legal nurse consultant. I have been a legal nurse consultant since 1987. For twenty years, I reviewed nursing malpractice cases and testified as an expert witness. In addition, since 1989, my company, Med League, has supplied expert witnesses for nursing and medical malpractice cases. I have heard the details of thousands of cases. The stories you will read in this book are all real occurrences. My own experiences as an expert witness are supplemented with published reports of lawsuits.

Table of Contents

Chapter 11 Tampering with Medical Records...............161

Chapter 12 Electronic Medical Records............167

Chapter 13 Summary..................................179

Chapter 1 Overview of Lawsuits

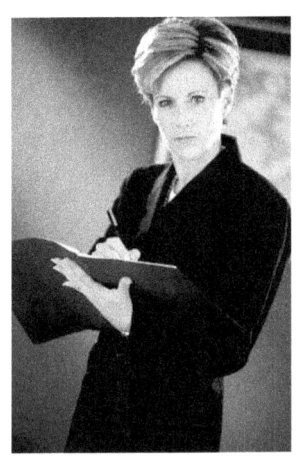

A forty-seven year-old man went to Community Medical Providers in May 2009 without a scheduled appointment. He complained of chest discomfort and indigestion-type symptoms. The staff requested that he go to Urgent Care, which took in walk-ins, but he wanted to be seen by his family physician. The doctor agreed to work him into the schedule when possible. The patient was placed in an exam room by the medical assistant. The medical assistant took vitals and discussed his symptoms. This information was given to the physician.

The medical assistant returned to the exam room about 40 minutes later and found the patient unconscious. Paramedics took him to the hospital, but the resuscitation effort failed.

The family of the man filed a lawsuit and alleged negligence in the failure to properly report the decedent's symptoms to the doctor, which would have led to a more prompt response by the doctor. The plaintiffs claimed that the staff should have been trained to recognize certain basic emergencies, and that the medical assistant should have appreciated that the decedent needed to be seen by a doctor right away.

The defendant claimed the decedent was suffering an acute coronary syndrome and that medical assistants in a family practice setting are not expected to triage patients as if they were in an urgent care or emergency setting.

Now that you have read this case, think about the role of the medical assistant. Is this person trained to recognize the patient's symptoms as an emergency? What do you think would have happened if an ambulatory care nurse assessed this patient, instead of a medical assistant? Do you think the outcome would have been different? Do you think the patient's actions had a role in the outcome?

This case went to trial. The jury did not find negligence. A defense verdict was returned. [1]

A lawsuit begins with an investigation of a concern by a patient or family member. The person who brings the suit is the plaintiff. The plaintiff may be the patient, or if he or she is not alive, the plaintiff may be a close family member.

The person or entity being sued is the defendant. After the plaintiff attorney reviews the facts of the case and decides that the case has merit, the attorney files a suit. In some states the attorney has the case reviewed by a healthcare professional of the same background as the defendant before filing suit. If this professional believes the case has merit, he or she files an affidavit of merit stating the case has merit. Filing the suit starts with a complaint that identifies the alleged deviations from the standard of care, the damages or injuries, and the demand for money.

The defense, once notified of the claim, reviews the complaint and formally responds to it. This begins the discovery phase. The plaintiff attorney is entitled to ask for documents, such as policies and procedures, job descriptions, and incident reports. Each side asks questions of the other, called interrogatories.

The plaintiff's deposition is taken, under oath in front of a court reporter, to gather information about what happened. The plaintiff is also usually asked how the injuries have affected his life. The depositions of the defendants, family members, and others with knowledge about the events are taken. The defendant doctors, nurses, and other healthcare professionals are asked questions under oath in front of a court reporter. The defendant's attorney prepares the professional for the types of questions that may be asked. Fact witnesses may also be deposed. These might be, for example, other nurses who worked in the healthcare setting with the defendant.

Each side hires expert witnesses to review the case to form their own opinions about the care that was provided. The use of expert witnesses, written reports and expert depositions varies greatly from state to state. In some states, the expert writes a report stating those opinions; each side provides the other with their expert reports. In almost all states, nursing expert witnesses (as opposed to physicians) evaluate the care of the nursing defendant. A physician expert is often used in a nursing malpractice case to determine if the injuries were caused by negligence. In many states, the expert prepares a report. In other states, the expert's opinions are outlined by the attorney in the form of a statement. In many states, the laws permit taking the deposition of the expert witness. This individual is questioned under oath by the attorney on the opposing side. The attorney evaluates the expert's demeanor, strength of conviction, and credibility.

Some cases are presented to a panel of reviewers before settlement or trial is discussed. Cases that have merit (with strong liability and injuries) are typically settled rather than the defense risking a large verdict if it is presented in court. The vast majority of cases settle.

Cases that go to court are either ones that the defense thinks are non-meritorious, or the amount of money the plaintiff has requested is out of proportion to what the defense and insurance carrier think is reasonable.

The case is heard by a judge ("a bench trial") or before a jury of 8-12 people. There are opening statements by both sides. The plaintiff's attorney goes first to present her case. The defendants and fact witnesses testify. They may be cross-examined (questioned by the opposing side's attorney). The expert witnesses testify as well.

The jury hears all of the evidence. In some courtrooms, they are allowed to take notes and even write out their own questions of a witness. After the plaintiff has finished presenting her case, the defense presents his case and calls witnesses. The attorneys may use exhibits in the courtroom to illustrate points and help the jury understand the medical issues of the case. The trial ends with closing statements by each attorney. Next, the judge explains the law to the jurors and the task before them in reaching a decision about the case. The jury goes to a room and discusses the case until they reach a verdict. The jury may award compensatory damages (money for the plaintiff). Rarely do they award punitive damages, which are designed to punish the defendant for behavior that is shocking. Punitive damages are not paid for by the insurance policy that your employer carries. Punitive damages are paid from the budget of the facility or wallet of the defendant.

The defense wins about 80% of the cases that go to trial. There are occasionally issues that arise during the trial that form the grounds for an appeal of the decision. At times, the defense appeals the size of a verdict.

Sometimes the attorneys reach an agreement that the names of the defendants and even the settlement amounts will be kept confidential.

The law in your state, the strategy of the attorneys, and the facts of a case may alter this typical pattern of a lawsuit. A suit may take 3-5 years to reach a conclusion.

Medical Malpractice Insurance

Many nurses ask me if they should have their own malpractice insurance policy. I recommend that nurses arrange for an insurance policy independent of their employer's coverage. There are three reasons for this.

1. Your activities as a nurse are not covered if you provide nursing care outside of your role as a nurse. If you give advice as a neighbor or friend, and that advice is negligent, you may be sued. Your employer's policy will not cover you as you were acting outside the scope of your employment.
2. Your employer's policy will not cover you if you are required to appear before the Board of Nursing for any reason. Your own insurance policy should provide you with representation from an attorney to represent you at the Board of Nursing hearings.
3. Policy premiums for nurses are relatively inexpensive, except for nurses working in high risk areas (such as labor and delivery) or high risk roles such as advanced practice nurses.

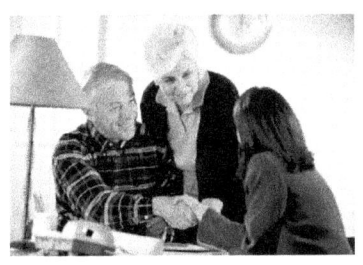

Chapter 2 Reasons People Sue

Why do people sue? Not everyone who is injured by a healthcare provider will seek the help of a plaintiff attorney. Many who do not sue are unaware of the negligence, forgive the healthcare provider, or do not want to undergo the rigors of a lawsuit. Less than 12% of people who are injured by malpractice file a lawsuit.

Desire for Answers

There are several reasons about why patients want to file a lawsuit against a healthcare provider. The reality is that most people seek out plaintiff attorneys to represent them because they want answers to what happened that led to a poor outcome. As healthcare providers, it is our legal and ethical responsibility to inform a patient and family about a negative outcome and what brought about that outcome. However, there are still healthcare professionals today who are just frankly scared to share information. They may provide a minimal or misleading explanation of what happened and why. Worst of all, they avoid and therefore anger the patient. However, a frank conversation about the outcome may possibly avert a suit.

Physicians are the people who are generally deemed responsible for explaining medical errors and untoward outcomes to patients. Some of them do it very well. Some of them are extraordinarily uncomfortable with the process and would rather be anywhere else than to sit in the patient's room and explain what happened. Physicians typically go into medicine because they want to help people, not harm them. They often feel guilty and inadequate when a patient is harmed.

Desire to Fix the System that Created the Error

Another subset of the people who contact plaintiff attorneys are motivated by a desire to make sure that the error that harmed them never happens to anybody else. They want to fix the system so that whatever caused the error will not recur. Unfortunately, the end result of a lawsuit is frequently limited to providing the plaintiff with financial compensation. It does not always result in changes in the system that caused the error. Even worse, healthcare providers do not always have a way to share lessons they have learned with other similar providers. The same errors are repeated.

Case Example

In a case that I reviewed as an expert witness, the plaintiff attorney was representing the estate of his cousin. The cousin had been a patient in a large Philadelphia hospital. On the day of discharge, he was complaining of leg pain and shortness of breath. The medical resident provided a phone discharge order without coming to the patient's bed to evaluate him. The nurse said, "What about the leg and the shortness of breath?" and the resident said, "Let him go." Twelve hours later, the patient dropped dead at home of a pulmonary embolism. His cousin, the plaintiff attorney, brought a suit. The case settled. One of the stipulations that was agreed to when it was settled was that this case would be taught to every resident and intern in the facility. The plaintiff attorney said, "Every July when you get that new group of people interns and residents, I want them to know about this." The hospital agreed that they would provide that education.

There are very few settlements that have conditions like this put in, but it would satisfy people a lot more if they knew not only why their loved one was harmed but as a result of that, they have changed something in the system. That's something plaintiffs desperately want.

Case Example
The plaintiff's decedent, age forty-nine, went to the emergency department at Kent Hospital in July 2006 with complaints of a burning pain in his throat, vomiting, and respiratory and pulse rates which were high. The decedent had previously had a stent placed in his chest. He was triaged as a less urgent patient, but a nurse sought to have a physician examine him. An EKG was performed, which was abnormal. The emergency room physician, Dr. Naylor, ordered cardiac monitoring. The monitoring was never initiated. The decedent was sent to the x-ray department and when he was returned to the emergency department, he was left on a gurney by a wall near a nurses' station. He suffered a fatal heart attack. There was a dispute between the parties as to whether or not the decedent was actually seen by a physician, with the decedent's fiancé, who was with him, testifying that he was not seen by a physician and Dr. Naylor and another physician both stating that they had seen the decedent. The defendants claimed that the decedent was appropriately treated for the symptoms he had and that nothing would have changed the outcome. The defendants specifically claimed that the EKG was not abnormal enough to warrant immediate action and that the computer's finding of "abnormal" was not conclusive. According to a published account, a confidential settlement was reached after the hospital's president apologized to the family. In addition to the payments to the plaintiffs, the hospital agreed to spend $1.25 million over the next five years for the Michael J. Woods Institute at Kent Hospital which will be charged with developing new procedures and training for the hospital's staff. The primary plaintiff in this case was actor James Woods, brother of the decedent, acting as

administrator for his brother's estate. The decedent's survivors included a minor's son.[2]

Desire for an Apology

Sometimes what people want is an apology and acknowledgement, such as, "We have made a mistake and we are sorry for what has happened." That is often not given. Many people in health care, in particular, are concerned that if they apologize that it will then come back to haunt them in a suit. There are several states that have "Sorry" laws. The law says, "If you apologize to a patient, then that information may not necessarily be shared with the jury at the time of a trial if that trial goes forward." The apology limits the number of people who will bring lawsuits because they have gotten what they wanted: an apology.

Case Example

I have a very good friend who was involved in a lawsuit with her mother. Her mother suffered several complications during surgery. The only thing my friend's family wanted was an apology. They were not there to make money. They didn't want the money. They ended up giving the money away, but they never got the apology, and that's really what they wanted. Learn more about this woman's story. Scan the QR code with your smart phone app.

Differing Expectations about Care

The result of cultural and personality differences is that patients have different expectations about the level of care that they're going to receive. The pressure of the healthcare environment and the staffing issues result in people not getting as much attention as they feel that they need. Of course, there is a degree of subjectivity when it comes to determining how much attention patients want. Some people who are stoics have been taught to not admit to a problem because they believe they are expected to just cope and not complain. There is the other extreme of the individuals who will, when you ask, "How are you?" will take it literally and tell you in detail. They can't get enough attention, and readily share their complaints.

High Pressured Care

Rapid turnover affects patient satisfaction. Patients are aware of decreased amount of time available to spend with doctors and nurses. Patients are aware of the pressures on clinics, hospitals, and doctors to provide rapid throughput: brief office visits and brief hospital admissions. To counter this pressure, there are some physicians who've come up with this idea of premium care. If you give them, for example, $5,000 a year to be your physician, the physician will promise that he or she will always be available to you. "I'll be on call; I'll come see you in the hospital; and I'll limit my patient load."

In a survey, when patients were asked what they thought causes the most medical errors, the number one reasons they cited were overwork, stress and the fatigue of healthcare professionals. The number two reason was doctors not having enough time with patients.

Some specialists are particularly prone to being sued based on the nature of their work. For example, orthopedic surgeons typically have a short timeframe to establish a rapport, develop a relationship, and do the surgery. When you don't have that personal connection with the doctor, it's easier to file a claim than it is against a family practice doctor who has been treating you for years.

Desire for Money

Some individuals will file a claim because of a desire for money. They've got medical bills they can't pay. A lot of individuals in our culture, unfortunately, don't have medical insurance and are looking for some source of funding to help pay for bills.

Health care has become very complex. We promise the public that we're going to take care of all of their concerns. Some hospitals advertise, "We provide the highest quality care." That's a statement that the plaintiff attorneys like to blow up in big letters for a courtroom exhibit. The attorney will cross examine the defendant and ask: "You promised the highest quality care but what did you deliver?"

In summary, patients turn to plaintiff attorneys when they want the satisfaction from understanding why the error occurred, to make a difference so the error that affected them will not hurt others, to get an apology, and to obtain money.

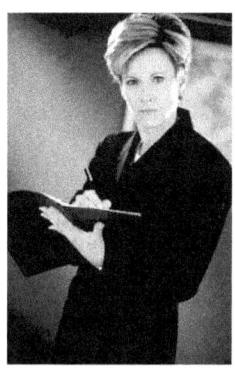

Chapter 3 Initial Steps in a Lawsuit

The Intake

Every lawsuit starts with contact with a plaintiff attorney. The first step is usually a phone call from the plaintiff. The plaintiff may be the patient if he or she is alive, or a family member with authority to act on behalf of a deceased patient.

The call is answered by a secretary, paralegal, nurse, or an attorney. There are several questions that are asked.

- What happened?
- Why do you think what occurred to you?
- What's your relationship to the person who was injured?
- Are there any injuries?
- Are they permanent?

Out of 100 phone calls that come in to a plaintiff attorney's office in a month, only a small number are investigated. It's about 5 cases. Many can be sorted out over the phone and rejected.

One of the first aspects of the case the attorney reviews is the damages or injuries to the patient. If the injuries are serious and permanent, the attorney next reviews other aspects of the case, including duty, breach of duty and proximate cause. These elements are described below.

For those cases that sound like they might have merit, the next step involves ordering and reviewing the medical records for those cases that are sorted out of the incoming calls. The plaintiff attorney will meet with the plaintiff. After discussing the facts of the case, the attorney makes a decision about whether to investigate the possible case.

Medical Record Review

The plaintiff attorney might request a copy of the chart or might ask the patient or family member to obtain it.

Once that chart has been handed over to the plaintiff attorney, any changes, alterations, additions, removals from that chart become detectable. Tampering with a medical record elevates the seriousness of the claim. Even if the defendant did nothing wrong, the case may become indefensible. Tampering with the record raises the risk of punitive damages being awarded at a trial. Tampering with a record can take what was a defensible case into a complicated and expensive case.

Recently a plaintiff attorney told me he settled a case after he discovered the staff tampered with the medical records. The patient was elderly. She was not resuscitated when her condition deteriorated. As he said, "She was going to die anyway, but when the staff altered the records, I was able to settle the case for $250,000, far more than it would have otherwise been worth."

Expert witness, legal nurse consultants, paralegals and attorneys review the medical records. They try to figure out the reasons the person needed care.

- What care was actually given?
- Was it given timely?
- Was it appropriate?

- What was the cause of the complication or the problem?

This is where the chart becomes crucial. Something that you wrote a year ago will be scrutinized. You never know whether that chart is indeed going to be something that will be reviewed in a plaintiff attorney's office.

What's in the chart is going to help or hurt the healthcare professional. In some cases it hurts the patient. For example, if the healthcare professional has documented the patient was advised to immediately go to the emergency department, and refused to do so, that documentation is going to be very helpful to the healthcare professional. I've worked with many attorneys who carefully look at notations of noncompliance. If some of the blame is going to be shifted to the plaintiff that affects how the case is going to be handled or if it's going to be filed at all.

Incident reports are typically available to the plaintiff attorney only after a case has been filed. Attorneys make assumptions that incident reports are written after untoward events, and will request the incident report after suit has been initiated.

Covering up an incident makes the case much harder to defend. The assumption is that the healthcare provider is trying to hide something and is acting in a guilty manner. Hiding an incident is far worse than acknowledging it.

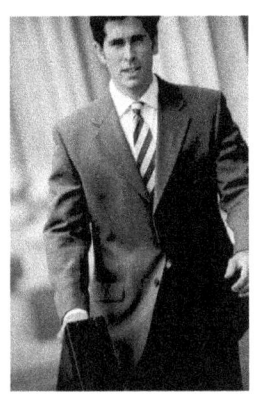

Chapter 4 Elements of Liability in an Ambulatory Nursing Malpractice Case

The plaintiff needs to establish that four elements were present at the time of the care:

- the nurse had a duty to the patient,
- the duty was breached or not followed,
- there were damages, and
- the actions of the healthcare provider were the proximate cause of the injuries.

Duty

The duty of the nurse to provide care is established through the relationship between the nurse and the patient. The nurse's relationship is created in many types of settings: hospital, nursing home, or other type of inpatient facility, home care, an ambulatory surgery setting, or similar outpatient facility. If the patient is in your facility, is on the grounds of your hospital, clinic or office, you have the duty to provide care and to follow the standards of care. If you're walking down the hospital hall and you see a patient trying to climb out of bed, you can't just say, "Not my patient, not my unit." You have to go in and say, "Wait a minute, can I give you some assistance or help?"

Case Example

Here is another example of examining the duty to care for a patient. An ambulance driver was taking a daughter and her mother to the hospital in an ambulance. Her daughter had a seizure at home. The driver encouraged the mother to come along in the ambulance to the hospital. The mother said, "I'm feeling faint. I don't really want to go." He said, "No, you need to be with your daughter." The mother got into the front of the ambulance in the seat next to the driver. They went to the hospital. When she got into the hospital, the mother felt faint. She fell and fractured her hip in the emergency department. The question from the plaintiff attorney to me was, "Did the ambulance attendant have a duty to help the mother get safely out of the ambulance and into the hospital?"

The daughter was the patient in the ambulance; the mother was not. The ambulance had a primary responsibility to the patient. You might say common courtesy would mean that he would help the mother get out of the vehicle, but she got out of the ambulance on her own; that was not when the fall occurred. She fell in the emergency department. So there was no duty between the attendant and the mother in that situation.

The attorney decided to reject the claim even though there were a lot of damages: the fractured hip, a lot of injury, a lot of debility, a lot of pain, and complications.

Breach of Duty/Standard of Care
The second element is a breach in the standard of care; something wasn't done correctly.

- Did the healthcare professional violate a policy?
- Was there a violation of a Joint Commission standard or a Department of Health regulation?
- Was it something that evidence based medical practice says that we should do?
- Are there authoritative (well respected) text books that say this is the way it should be done?

The standards of care are used to define the breaches in the performance of the nurse. Standards are based on nursing literature, professional association standards, such as the American Academy of Ambulatory Care Nursing, common practice, and evidence based research. The standards of care are also defined in practice guidelines, institutional policies and procedures, governmental regulations, Joint Commission standards, state practice acts, and so on. The attorney and expert witnesses evaluate whether there was a clear cut breach from the standard of care.

Simple errors in judgment or bad outcomes do not necessarily equate to medical malpractice or nursing malpractice. Somebody has to do something wrong. That's not always clear, because there are a couple of different ways that you can accomplish your objectives. You can get a patient to the bathroom with one person or with two people. You can make a decision in the situation that it's safe to use one person to take the patient to the bathroom. You don't anticipate that the patient was going to feel faint part way to the bathroom.

If you make a reasonable judgment in the situation, but then it turns out wrong, that's not necessarily a breach of the standard of care. But suppose you say to the patient, "Oh, I know you're feeling dizzy, but it will clear. Come on, let's go." When you ignore the warning signs that could be considered a breach in judgment or a breach in the standard of care.

There are lots of cases that I have been involved in related to this issue. Was what happened to the patient a foreseeable outcome? Assume the patient is in the bathroom and is told, "Don't get off the toilet until I come back to help you." Is it foreseeable that that patient is going to get up on her own and fall and fracture her ankle? Somebody who is reasonably alert and is able to follow instructions would not make you suspect that she would get up on her own.

Case Example
I testified in a case involving a very experienced nurse who was a former Director of Nursing of the Operating Room. She was a patient in the hospital and even though she was told repeatedly, "Don't get up off the toilet without asking for assistance", she got up on her own. She was overconfident and not easily directed. She fell and fractured her ankle.

I testified on behalf of the hospital that if she had been given this instruction, it was reasonable for the aide to expect the patient would follow the direction. The aide stood outside the bathroom door. She was within an arm's reach of the doorknob and would've been able to hear this patient saying, "Can you give me some help?" She was right there, but the woman decided to get up on her own and fell. The defense won the case.

Damages
The third element is injury. There has to be some kind of injury. Injuries are usually the first element that a plaintiff attorney will evaluate. Attorneys typically evaluate the damages in a case before examining other elements, such as duty, breach of duty or proximate cause. There must be damages or injuries, either psychological or physical, as a result of the breach in care. Few plaintiff attorneys are interested in representing patients who have only

psychological or emotional damages, although there are exceptions.

Experienced attorneys don't get involved in cases that have minor damages, temporary injuries, or no residual effects. Those cases are really not worthwhile spending $100,000 or more to take through the litigation process. Plaintiff attorneys carefully evaluate the big injury cases and they look for cases where somebody was relatively healthy, not somebody who was likely to have died from another possible reason.

Brain injuries, spinal cord injuries, and birth injuries are examples of high damages cases. The injury should be substantial, not that the patient was dissatisfied with the quality of care, or that a staff member did not respond fast enough or the hospital food was terrible.

The plaintiff attorney considers the age and earning capability of the patient. The attorney also considers whether the patient had dependents. The case of a middle aged man who had a good paying job is worth more than that of a child, for example.

Causation
The last element is causation. Was there a link between what the ambulatory care nurse did and the outcome? The actions of the nurse must be the proximate cause of the injury. A bad outcome may occur in the absence of negligence. We know that health care can result in terrible outcomes. People die, bleed, get infections, or fall. Is there a link between what the nurse did and the injury? If there is not a link, this is going to be the element that will destroy the case. All four of these pieces have to be in place for the plaintiff to win.

A Nice Plaintiff

There is a fifth important element, which is an informal one. If the patient is not a nice person, then the jury is not going to give him money. The jury should be able to identify with the plaintiff. Individuals with a criminal background or substance abuse problems, for example, may not prove to be attractive plaintiffs. As one plaintiff attorney said, "Ask yourself if you would fly across the country sitting next to the plaintiff. If the answer is 'no', think twice about representing them."

Case Example

To give you an example of this, I evaluated a case as an expert witness that involved a woman who was in an urban hospital. She was a substance abuser. She came in because she had deep vein thrombosis. She was wandering around the hospital halls, and the nurses were not really paying attention to the reason for her wandering. They told her to go back to her room but she did not return to her room.

The patient was searching. No one understood what she was doing and no one was paying attention. She went into a hallway where she found an unlocked medication cart. She pulled open the drawers and she found syringes. Now this is something that's like gold if you are a drug addict. She found a 30 cc vial of Lasix and a 30 cc vial of insulin. She injected herself with the contents of both vials. Why? Clearly she wasn't thinking correctly.

The Lasix was not harmful, but the whole vial of insulin caused her blood sugar to go down. When she was found seizing, she had a blood sugar of about 5. She damaged her brain. Ironically, before this, she was a real problem for her family because she was always on the street trying to get drugs. She was unable to care for her child; the grandmother took care of the child. After her brain injury, she became very docile and easy to manage.

Let's consider the 4 elements of a valid medical malpractice suit. Did the nurses have a duty to observe her and to keep the cart locked? Did they breach their duty by leaving the cart unlocked in the hallway? Did she become injured, and was there a link between the actions of the nurses and the injury? The answer to all of these questions, in my opinion, was "yes".

The trial took place in an urban city. It took two days for the jury to be picked. One of the questions the judge asked was, "Do you think that an IV drug user is entitled to the same standard of care as anyone else?" Potential jurors kept saying "no".

At the end of two days, the judge finally had eight people who could answer "yes." In reality, the jury agreed that all of the four elements were present. But this plaintiff was not nice and they gave her no money at all. I think they wondered what would happen if they awarded her money. They probably envisioned the patient getting high with the money.

This was the first medical malpractice case the plaintiff attorney ever took. He told me it's also the very last medical malpractice case that he will take. Most plaintiff attorneys would not accept a case like that because of her substance abuse problem.

Sometimes the judge will say, "The jury is not entitled to know that negative information about the patient" but in this case, there was no way to prevent the jury from knowing about this woman's substance abuse problem. Her drug seeking was a critical element in the case.

Case Example
Joe was a man who was an IV drug user who became paralyzed when he was intoxicated. He was not sure whether he got hit by a train or a car. He became paralyzed and he was in a nursing home. He had a very foul mouth. He swore at the aides. One day, he asked the aide if she would give him a bath. He said, "The water is not hot enough. Can you get hotter water?" Remember, he had no feeling from his waist to his toes. The aide went to the coffee urn and she got hot water. It was later tested at 180 degrees.

When I met Joe in the burn unit, he said, "I sat there and I watched the water turn brown and little strips of skin came floating to the surface of the water." He ended up with such severe scalding that his legs were amputated as a way to try to control his condition. He survived for about a year before he died; this was before the trial.

Joe's case met the four elements of liability. But he was not a particularly nice person and the defense attorneys really played that up at trial. The plaintiff attorney thought that the case was worth probably a million dollars or so. He made an agreement with the defense attorney by saying, "If the jury gives any money at all, then the low amount that I will accept is $900,000, and if they give any money at all, the high amount that I will hold you to is 1.5 million." This is called a high-low agreement. The jury came back and awarded Joe's family $120,000. Under the high-low agreement, the award was raised to $900,000. Had Joe lived, his case would have been worth more because of the care he needed.

Statute of Limitations

In each state, there is a statute of limitations or the allowable time to start a lawsuit. For example, if your state has a 2 year statute of limitations, the plaintiff has 2 years from the time that he knew or should have known there was a medical error.

Case Example

For example, a patient has an abdominal surgery, and somebody leaves behind an abdominal pad, a lap pad, a towel, or a clamp. The patient is sewn up without anyone detecting that. A year later he is finally diagnosed after having abdominal adhesions and abdominal pain. In a case that I worked on recently, the sponge actually worked its way up towards the skin and the doctor felt a hard lump under the skin.

When the patient realized the pad was inside, the statute of limitations began. When he knew or he should have known he had the lap pad in his abdomen from his surgery a year ago, that's when the clock start ticking, not from the original surgery date. Childbirth cases are a bit different. The child has 18 years plus 2 years to file suit, in most states.

The Nursing Process

Most, if not all, deviations from the nursing standard of care are rooted in omitting or improperly carrying out one of the steps of the nursing process. Nurses provide care based on the nursing process. We:

- assess the needs of the patient,
- formulate nursing diagnoses,
- develop a plan of care,
- implement the plan, and
- evaluate its effectiveness.

Resources on the Nursing Process

Obtain a copy of the state nurse practice act. Many of the practice acts are based on the nursing process. Many of the standards of practice published by the American Nurses Association are based on the nursing process.

Several cases involving nursing liability revolve around a failure to carry out one or more steps of the nursing process. Nursing liability cases may also reveal weaknesses in the way care is delivered or broader systemic issues that deal with inadequate equipment, miscommunication, delays in delivering care and other issues. Ideally, lessons learned as a result of a patient injury or lawsuits are transmitted to others within the system so that the system can be examined to see what kinds of improvements are needed.

Chapter 5 Allegations

The majority of nursing negligence cases that are reported in the legal literature focus on nurses employed by hospitals, since they represent the largest nursing labor force. However, no nurse is immune from participating in care that results in an untoward outcome or a disgruntled patient. This text includes summaries of cases in different health care settings. Although you are an ambulatory care nurse, read the case to apply the principles to your setting.

A study of case reports revealed that many of the allegations against nurses tend to fall within one of several categories:

- Failure to follow the standards of care.
- Failure to use equipment in a responsible manner.
- Failure to communicate.
- Failure to document.
- Failure to assess and monitor.
- Failure to act as a patient advocate. [3]

1. Failure to Follow the Standards of Care

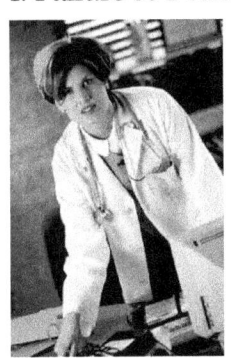
Failure to follow the standards of care covers a broad range of behaviors and is based on an analysis of what the reasonably prudent nurse would do in the same or similar situation. Nursing standards of care are based on nursing education, publications, and state and federal standards. The ultimate goal is to protect patients. The multiple goals of nursing care include providing a safe environment; restoring and maintaining the highest level of functional independence as possible; preserving autonomy, and stabilizing and delaying the progression of chronic

medical problems. The nursing staff is intimately involved in helping to achieve these goals. In order to do so, standards of care must be followed.

The legal team evaluates a claim based on the standards of care in effect at the time that care was given. Ambulatory care nurses are guided by the Telehealth Nursing Practice Administration and Practice Standards published by American Academy of Ambulatory Care Nursing [4] as well as position statements such as "The Role of the Registered Nurse in Ambulatory Care". [5]

Here is an example of a case in which the plaintiff alleged a failure to follow the standards of care.

Case Example
The plaintiff's decedent, age seventy-two, went to the defendant's walk in clinic with complaints of persistent coughing and shortness of breath. She was diagnosed with acute bronchitis and was instructed to return to the clinic if her symptoms did not respond to the antibiotics which were prescribed. The decedent returned with her daughter the next week. The decedent had similar complaints. A chest x-ray was normal. The decedent was diagnosed with likely respiratory illness and referred to a pulmonologist. She went home and suffered a massive heart attack the next day.

The plaintiff claimed that an EKG should have been ordered and that the decedent should have been referred for a cardiac evaluation. The defendant argued that the decedent denied chest pain and angina symptoms during the evaluation and that the diagnosis made was reasonable. [6]

Feedback Question
Based on the above case, define the standard of care the plaintiff alleged was not followed. Who do you think won

the case?

Answer
The standard of care is to protect the patient from injury and to correctly diagnose her condition. The defense won this case. The symptoms were not indicative of a cardiac origin. A nurse might be named as a defendant in a failure to diagnose case if the nurse inaccurately recorded symptoms.

The material included in this section focuses on the responsibilities of both the nurse and the nursing administration. Although the nurse's actions are often most highly exposed when an injury occurs, the nurse does not function in a vacuum. Decisions made by the management of the facility, unit, office practice or clinic impact the nurse's practice.

Feedback Question
What are the responsibilities of the nursing administration related to the nursing standards of care?

Answer
The nursing administration responsibilities include:

- Ensure that the nursing standards of care are incorporated into policies and procedures. Update policies with evidence-based literature to ensure the standards are current.
- Integrate the standards of the American Academy of Ambulatory Care Nursing into the facility's standards.
- Participate in planning sessions with the education department to ensure that the educational needs of the staff are identified and addressed.
- Support sending staff to clinical conferences to learn more about changes in nursing practice, update

knowledge and skills, and to bring the information back to the staff.

Ambulatory care nurses who work in Joint Commission accredited facilities are also expected to be aware of the National Patient Safety Goals. The four 2012 goals focus on:

- Identifying patients correctly
- Using medicines safely
- Preventing infection
- Preventing mistakes in surgery [7]

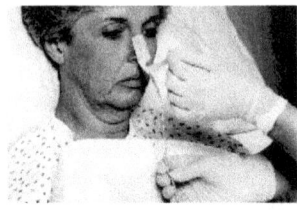

2. Failure to Use Equipment in a Responsible Manner

A huge variety of medical equipment is used in the care of patients. Foley catheter tubes, feeding tubes, ventilators, assistive devices for walking, physical therapy splints and tubs, side rails, wheelchairs, intravenous catheters, dialysis catheters and others can all be misused. Nurses have a duty to exercise reasonable care in the use of medical equipment. They are expected to understand how to safely operate equipment.

The *Top Ten Health Technology Hazards for 2012* report issued by ECRI identified equipment hazards. Many of these hazards are related to equipment used in ambulatory care. The hazards are:

1. Alarm hazards
2. Exposure hazards from radiation therapy and CT
3. Medication administration errors using infusion pumps
4. Cross-contamination from flexible endoscopes

5. Inattention to change management for medical device connectivity
6. Enteral feeding misconnections
7. Surgical fires
8. Needle stick and other sharps injuries
9. Anesthesia hazards due to incomplete pre-use inspection
10. Poor usability of home-use medical devices [8]

Cross contamination occurs from improperly reprocessed flexible endoscopes. Contamination can cause life-threatening infections at worst and at best, detrimental to a facility's reputation and causes patient anxiety when they are told they may have been exposed to a contaminated endoscope. Reprocessing requires constant adherence to a multistep procedure of cleaning.

Often, devices that are used in the home were not designed with the lay user in mind. They are frequently very difficult to use and may there be inadequate patient training. The devices may lack labeling or instructions for use or maintenance.

Surgical fires occur 600 times a year in the US. Virtually all fires can be avoided.

Needle stick injuries can result in the healthcare provider being exposed to hepatitis, HIV, and other infections.

Feedback Question
What are the responsibilities of the nurse related to the use of equipment?

Answer

The nurse is expected to know how to safely use equipment, and to seek assistance when faced with unfamiliar equipment.

Feedback Question

What are the responsibilities of the nurse manager related to the use of equipment?

Answer

The nurse manager's responsibilities include:

- Ensure that inservice education is provided when a new piece of equipment is placed into use in the work environment.
- Ensure that manuals for equipment are located in an area accessible to all who need the information.
- Ensure there is a mechanism for nurses who miss the educational sessions to obtain the information about the new equipment.
- Advise staff to notify the appropriate person if there are concerns about the functioning of equipment.
- Retain the equipment after a patient injury has occurred so that the equipment may be examined. Destruction of the equipment may be construed as tampering with evidence.

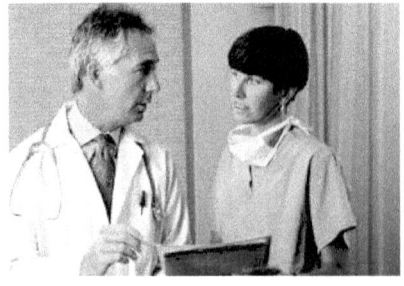

3. Failure to Communicate
According to the Joint Commission, communication has been found to be the number one contributor to patient injury. In today's

multicultural society, sources of misunderstanding and miscommunication can result in multiple opportunities for errors resulting in harm to patients. Communication barriers between patients and nurses, and nurses and other healthcare workers can result in inappropriate orders, incorrect interventions or failure to take action. Absence of communication also sets up a climate for errors to occur.

Lack of communication may convey lack of interest, concern, leadership, or knowledge. Communication is the glue that holds a team together. Examples of communication gaps that may influence patient safety are shown below.

Samples of Communication Contributors to Patient Injury

- The patient calling the telehealth line speaks no English, and the telehealth nurse is unable to determine what language he speaks.
- A patient's explanation of symptoms may be misinterpreted by a nurse with limited knowledge of English.
- The patient does not report one of the symptoms he is having because he does not think it is significant.
- The patient cannot give a good history; she is a "poor historian".
- The medical practice has no system in place to follow up with patients who miss appointments.
- A female nurse who comes from a culture of subservient women may be reluctant to question a male doctor who writes an incorrect order.
- Policy and procedure manuals are stored on an inaccessible shelf and are often out of date, not reflecting current practice.

- A stoic nurse who minimizes the patient's pain can delay reporting an ominous development of chest pain.
- The medical practice fails to notify a patient of an abnormal test result, which needs follow up.
- There is no mechanism for an employee to make a suggestion to correct a safety problem, and no recognition for such ideas.
- An abusive physician is permitted to publicly chastise nurses because he brings a large volume of patients into the hospital. [9]

Case Example

Consider the miscommunication associated with this case.

The plaintiff underwent a chest x-ray in October 2001 as part of his mandatory annual comprehensive medical examination as a firefighter. The chest x-ray revealed a small nodular density in the left upper lobe that appeared larger as compared to previous chest x-rays since 1996. The radiologist correctly recommended a chest CT scan to rule out lung cancer, but this information was never conveyed to the plaintiff. In August 2005, the plaintiff was diagnosed with Stage IIIA lung cancer which had spread and was given a five-year, ten percent survival rate.

Discovery revealed that the nurse who gathered the test results of the physical examination in October 2001 mistakenly provided this physician with the chest x-ray report from the previous year, which had been read as normal. The plaintiff claimed that if the correct report had been provided to the physician, a work up for lung cancer would have occurred in October 2001; which would have led to diagnosis of Stage IA lung cancer, which would have been curable. The plaintiff also claimed negligence by the physician in not noting that the chest x-ray report was from August 2000, not October 2001. The plaintiff also claimed that the radiologist who interpreted the August 2000 chest x-ray had failed to appreciate that the lesion was slightly larger on that x-ray as compared to chest x-rays obtained in 1998 and 1996.

In October 2004, the plaintiff was scheduled for lumbar surgery and preoperative chest x-rays were ordered, which were properly interpreted as showing an upper lobe nodule suspicious for neoplasm. That radiologist recommended a chest CT for further evaluation. The radiologist noted that this information was forwarded by phone to the neurosurgeon's office and the written report was subsequently sent to the neurosurgeon, who initialed the report as having been reviewed. The neurosurgeon, however, did not inform the plaintiff of the abnormal chest x-ray findings.

The neurosurgeon testified that he did not receive the message from the radiologist and that he had not actually reviewed the written report, even though he initialed it, because the written report arrived after the surgery had been performed. The physician who received the wrong report in October 2001 claimed that it was reasonable for him to rely on the nurse. The radiologist who interpreted the August

2000 x-ray contended that the interpretation of the chest x-ray had been proper. According to a published account, a $1.7 million settlement was reached, which included the future wrongful death claim. [10]

Feedback Question
How many people miscommunicated in this example?

Answer
At a minimum, the nurse and the neurosurgeon miscommunicated.

Feedback Question
What are the responsibilities of the nurse related to miscommunication?

Answer
The nurse is responsible for:

- Identifying and reporting concerning changes in the patient's condition.
- Repeating back telephone and verbal orders to confirm that they have been properly heard.
- Asking individuals to repeat back understanding of what has been said, for example, during patient education.
- Acting as part of a multidisciplinary team to encourage collaboration and mutual respect for the contributions of each discipline. Costly teamwork failures need to be avoided, such as:
  - Failure to identify an established protocol for patient care or even to develop a treatment plan.
  - Failure to advocate and assert an alternative plan or corrective course of action when a question arises about the patient's care.
  - Failure to prioritize caregiver tasks for the patient.
  - Failure to cross-monitor actions of other team members. [11]

Feedback Question
What are the responsibilities of the nurse manager related to miscommunication?

Answer

The nurse manager's responsibilities include:

- Ensure that a translator service is available for use in the care of patients.
- Encourage staff to speak up when they do not understand what another person is saying.
- Encourage staff from different shifts to work together to resolve issues that affect the smooth functioning of the nursing unit.
- Assist staff to recognize that communication skills decrease during stress and fatigue, and that extra caution needs to be employed during those vulnerable times.

More on communication is presented in the section below on delay of treatment.

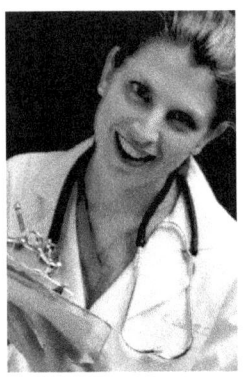

4. Failure to Document

Documentation is part of the nurse's overall responsibility for patient care. The clinical record facilitates care, enhances continuity of care, and helps coordinate the treatment and evaluation of the patient. One of the most significant professional functions of the registered nurse is the evaluation of the patient's responses to nursing care.

Professional nurses are responsible for managing increasingly complex patient issues and coordinating patient care among many levels of healthcare workers. Documentation must clearly communicate a nurse's judgment and evaluation of the patient's status. [12]

Review the case below and identify how documentation affected the outcome.

Case Example

The plaintiff, in his seventies, was admitted to the defendant hospital in July 2003 for a transurethral resection of the prostate (TURP) by defendant urologist Dr. Zamora. After the procedure, Dr. Zamora set up a continuous bladder irrigation (CBI) to prevent blood clots. The next morning the plaintiff's bladder ruptured, leading to kidney failure, respiratory failure, infections and a two-month hospitalization. The plaintiff claimed that he could no longer drive a car due to the incident. The plaintiff claimed that the hospital's nurses failed to monitor and document the fluid intake and output during the CBI, which led to the bladder rupture. The plaintiff claimed that Dr. Zamora used water for irrigation instead of saline, which caused hyponatremia and that Dr. Zamora failed to order the nurses to document fluid intake and output during the CBI. The defendants claimed that there was no negligence.

According to a published account a jury returned a verdict against the hospital, but in favor of Dr. Zamora. The verdict was $1,531,000. The damages, however, were capped and the plaintiffs received a total of $397,716. Appeals were expected. [13]

Documentation Practices

A nursing malpractice case will be decided in part on how well the nurse has documented in the medical record. A clearly written record which explains the care that was delivered will avert many lawsuits. This is a quick overview of charting guidelines. Documentation is covered in greater depth later in this book.

Charting should:

- Be clearly written using correct grammar and spelling.
- Be timely - written as close to the delivery of care as possible and practical.
- Be focused on the patient's primary needs.
- Be individualized to the needs of the patient.
- Clearly identify changes in the patient's condition, and the steps that were taken, as appropriate, to report changes to the primary care provider-physician, nurse practitioner or physician's assistant.
- Not have obliterations or erasures. Instead, a mistaken entry should be identified with the original entry still readable.
- Be free of unauthorized abbreviations and avoid using the ones associated with high risk for misinterpretation, such as U for units, IU for international units, QD and QOD, MS04 and MgS04, and others specific to the clinical area.
- Carefully document reading back and verification of phone or verbal orders.
- Record what the nurse did to report critical lab results or changes in the patient's condition, including the name of the person who was informed and the action that was taken as a result.
- Verify that a time out was performed to identify the right patient, right site, and right procedure before an invasive procedure is performed.
- Contain accurate counts of surgical instruments, sharps, and sponges and record what was done if the count was inaccurate.

- Verify that alarms are set on equipment.
- Contain a complete list of the patient's medications when the patient is transferred from one site of care to another or upon admission to a facility.
- Contain accurate fall risk assessments.
- Contain pressure ulcer risk assessments on admission to a facility and periodically thereafter.
- Record the sites used to give intramuscular or subcutaneous injections.
- Identify patients at risk for committing suicide, and detail the plan of care needed to protect them.
- Contain an updated care plan that is individualized to the patient.
- Be free of words that convey bias or dislike, such as "sloppy", "drunk", "obnoxious", and so on.
- Verify the patient in restraints was frequently observed, offered food or fluid, the restraints were released, and the rationale for the use of restraints, as per state and federal regulations.
- Identify allergies.
- Record any noncompliance by the patient or family, and the results of efforts by the nursing staff to inform the patient of the consequences of noncompliance.
- Be free of criticism of other healthcare providers.
- Verify that assessments were performed.
- Detail the reason why medications or other care was omitted.
- Not be done before care is rendered.
- Be entered into the correct chart.
- Contain specific times when care was rendered.
- Be legible.
- Be comprehensive.
- Not be destroyed.

- Be dated and timed with the patient's name on every sheet in the medical record.
- Contain, if necessary, clearly identified late entries added on the next available line.
- Contain the patient's words when describing symptoms.
- Utilize a pain scale, whenever possible, to record the level of pain before and after interventions designed to reduce the pain.
- Signed with the nurse's name and title.
- Be devoid of spaces that would permit someone else to enter information into the nurse's note.
- Not be placed in an area where it is accessible to the patient, family, or visitors.

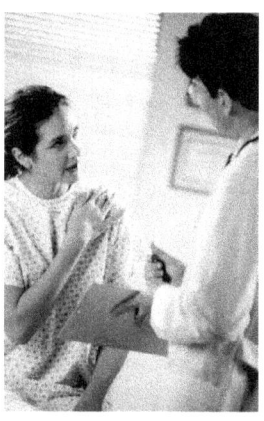

5. Failure to Assess and Monitor
The American Nurses Association standard for assessment includes measurement criteria that focus on the following: The registered nurse:

- Collects data in a systematic and ongoing process.
- Involves the patient, family, other healthcare providers, and environment, as appropriate, in holistic data collection.
- Prioritizes data collection activities based on the patient's immediate condition, or anticipated needs of the patient or situation.
- Uses appropriate evidence-based assessment techniques and instruments in collecting pertinent data.
- Uses analytical models and problem-solving tools.

- Synthesizes available data, information, and knowledge relevant to the situation to identify patterns and variances.[14]

Case Example

The plaintiff, age fifty-three, arrived at Mazzocco Ambulatory Surgery Center for placement of a prosthetic lens in his left eye. The plaintiff suffered from diabetes and a serious kidney disease. The plaintiff claimed that after anesthesiologist Phillip Spiegel administered anesthesia, he left the room. The patient was monitored by nursing staff with inadequate training in monitoring sedated patients. The plaintiff claimed that he suffered a reaction to the anesthesia, resulting in a deeper state of sedation and subsequently sustained a blocked airway. He had a respiratory arrest that went unnoticed for several minutes. The plaintiff suffered severe anoxic brain damage and is confined to a skilled nursing center. The plaintiff settled with Dr. Spiegel for a confidential amount prior to trial. The case proceeded to trial against the surgery center. The jury returned a $2,245,000 verdict. [15]

Astute assessment is needed to detect problems and changes in the patient's condition. These changes should be communicated by the registered nurse to the clinical decision maker - whether that is a physician, nurse practitioner, or physician's assistant. Many legal cases revolve around the issues of changes in the patient's condition, and whether anyone was notified of the concerns.

In the following case, the clinic employees deviated from the standard of care regarding assessments.

Case Example
The plaintiff's decedent went to the defendant clinic in July 2007 and saw the defendant doctor with complaints of various body pains. There were no notes made in the medical record that a physical exam was performed or that a medical history was taken. Two days later the decedent was found dead in his bed. An autopsy report found the death to be due to an accidental overdose of the prescribed narcotics. The plaintiff claimed that the defendants had been negligent in prescribing narcotics without medical necessity and alleged that the defendants were running a "pill mill" in routinely prescribing narcotic medications without a proper exam. The defendant denied any negligence and alleged that the decedent had failed to take the narcotics as prescribed. The jury found the defendant doctor, the clinic, and the partners in the clinic all negligent. Fault was apportioned sixty-five percent to the defendant doctor, thirty-five percent to the clinic and five percent to the partners. A $2,438,260 verdict was returned. [16]

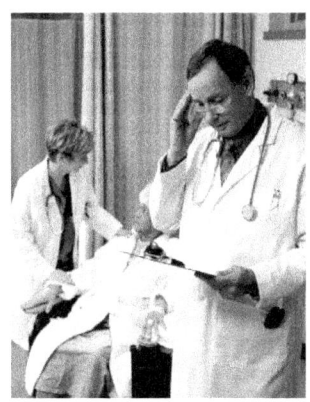

6. Failure to Act as a Patient Advocate
The nurse is expected to protect patients. This obligation flows from standards of professional practice and the American Nurses Association's Code of Ethics for Nurses (2010). Statement 3 says: "The nurse promotes, advocates and strives to protect the health, safety, and rights of the patient."

1. The nurse safeguards the patient's right to privacy and confidentiality.

2. The patient has a right to choose if he wants to participate in research.

3. The nurse has the responsibility to implement and maintain standards of professional practice.

4. As an advocate for the patient, the nurse must be alert to and take appropriate action regarding any instances of incompetent, unethical, illegal, or impaired practice by any member of the health care team or the healthcare system or any action of others that places the rights or best interests of the patient in jeopardy.

Failure to act as a patient advocate or go up the chain of command for a patient can lead to nursing malpractice suits. Patients, even the most informed, run into difficulties figuring out how to navigate the complexities of the healthcare environment. They call nurses seeking help. The nursing advocacy role is high in the telehealth environment. Patients count on nurses to help them obtain the needed care. The nurses they call should understand the system, how to access it, and what is available. In some cases, nurses must be prepared to act on the patient's behalf. At times, the nurse has to step in for the patient who is not acting in his best interest, or is unable to act. This may mean sending an ambulance to the house, for example.

Failing to act as a patient advocate encompasses the responsibility to protect the patient from harm by actively promoting safety and challenging others' orders. The chain of command is the mechanism used within a facility or practice area to provide employees with a process for resolving clinical or administrative concerns. When the concern is related to a patient, and cannot be resolved by the nursing manager/supervisor, the physician chain of command may be invoked. The attending physician or department head may become involved in resolving the issue. The chain of command is variable depending on the setting.

Chain of command policy should cover these points:

- A policy that is individualized to the facility should be defined in writing.
- The policy should be easy to understand and implement.
- There should be a statement that all staff is responsible for using the chain of command when there is a patient care concern.
- The policy should contain some examples of when the chain of command should be used, such as:
  - A physician has not responded in a timely fashion to the deterioration of a patient's condition.
  - A healthcare provider is suspected of being impaired by chemicals, alcohol, extreme fatigue or other factors.
  - A prescriber's orders are unclear and the prescriber cannot clarify them.
  - The nurse's assessment of the patient is markedly different from the physician's.
  - In a clinical situation when the nurse believes the prescriber has not fully responded to issues that may pose an immediate risk to the patient.

The policy should:

- Detail the specific steps to be taken and the job titles to be contacted and the order in which they should be contacted.

- Include pointers on how to document the situation, if applicable, in the patient's medical record.
- Instruct staff to avoid name calling or making general statements of dissatisfaction with the situation, facility, or provider, in the medical record.
- Specify that there will be no retaliation against an employee who invokes the chain of command policy.

Nurse managers should:

- Ensure that prescribers are aware of nursing administration's support of its employees.
- Encourage staff to express their concerns related to a provider who is performing below standard.
- Actively use the chain of command to carry the concerns of clinical staff to the appropriate medical or administrative person.
- Provide education regarding the use of the chain of command policy. [17]

If the nurse manager fails to inform the physician/prescriber of a clinical concern that warrants the use of the chain of command, the manager may be liable.

The nurse manager may be the recipient of concerns from staff nurses who are questioning orders. The nurse manager should first talk over the situation with the physician; if that does not resolve the concern, the chain of command within the facility should be used. [18] Nurses are being held accountable if they carried out an order that they knew was harmful to the patient, or were not active enough in getting the order changed.

Case Example

The plaintiff's decedent underwent surgery to insert an aortic valve graft in March 1998. He had no post-operative complications and was discharged after three days with Coumadin and Heparin. He had trouble at home keeping his coagulation in the correct range, so he was readmitted to the hospital three days later to regulate his blood levels. After nine days, the records indicated that the levels were appropriate and he was to be discharged the next day. In the very early morning hours of the discharge day, the decedent experienced a sudden onset of pain between his shoulder blades, into his back and chest. He walked to the nurse's station and reported this to the defendant nurse and requested to be seen by a doctor.

The nurse checked his vital signs, which were reportedly normal and called the defendant physician's assistant. Over the telephone the physician's assistant instructed the nurse to give the decedent pain medication and take him back to bed. The decedent continued to complain of severe back pain and repeatedly asked the defendant nurse to help him. The nurse gave him pain medication and a sedative, and called the defendant nursing supervisor to come see him. The defendant nursing supervisor found the decedent agitated, in a lot of pain and begging for someone to help him. The nursing supervisor gave him a back rub and assured him he would be fine.

Twenty minutes after he began complaining of the pain the decedent became diaphoretic, indicated that the pain was crossing through his chest and continued to ask for help. Within two minutes he suffered cardiopulmonary arrest and a code was called. He was not able to be resuscitated. The medical examiner who conducted the autopsy indicated that death was probably caused by a cardiac arrhythmia as a result of the valve surgery. The plaintiff claimed that the defendants were negligent in failing to summon a physician to evaluate the decedent and in failing to place him on an EKG monitor. The plaintiff claimed that the EKG would have shown an abnormal heart rhythm which could have been treated.

The defendants claimed that there was no negligence and that all vital signs were normal, showing him to be in no immediate danger. The defendants also claimed that the decedent died of a sudden cardiac event unrelated to his initial back pain. According to a published account, a $2 million settlement was reached. [19]

Feedback Question
What was the role of the nursing supervisor in this case, and did the supervisor fulfill the standards of care and act as an advocate for the patient?

Answer
The nursing supervisor failed to recognize the signs of deterioration and delayed seeking treatment for the patient.

Case Example
As many as 115 patients may have contracted hepatitis as a result of the reuse of single use items in two clinics in Nevada. The 2008 investigation showed that nurses reused syringes, medication vials, bite blocks and other equipment intended for single use. Twenty two RNs and LPNs were investigated in connection to the hepatitis outbreak. Several are still under investigation by the Nevada Board of Nursing for alleged violations that included failure to safeguard a patient, failure to properly document, falsification of medical records, and failure to conform to customary standards of practice.

Dr. Lisa Black performed a study of Nevada nurses' attitudes towards being patient advocates and the factors that held them back from reporting unsafe practices. She found that 34% of her sample (564 people returned the survey) indicated they were aware of a patient care condition that could have caused harm to a patient, yet had not reported it. The most common reasons for non-reporting included fear of workplace retaliation and a belief that nothing would come of reports that were made. [20]

Nurses are obligated to be patient advocates, to protect the vulnerable, to speak out on the patient's behalf, to question inappropriate orders and practices. Yet they sometimes hold back. There are numerous consequences in some settings for speaking out.

- Demotion
- Pressure to resign
- Referral to mental health providers
- Fear of losing one's job
- Belief concerns will be ignored
- Fear of retaliation

The fear that concerned employees will not risk the consequences of speaking out, or blowing the whistle, has led many states to put laws into place to protect employees from punishment. The laws vary from state to state.

Feedback Question
What can you do *as a patient* if you are aware that a nurse is questioning something about your care?

Answer
Find out what the nurse is concerned about. Ask for details. Ask for an explanation of what could happen to you if the

safety concern is not corrected. Encourage that nurse to speak out. Realize that the nurse's loyalty to his or her employer may silence the nurse. If you are in a position to seek care elsewhere, get yourself out of the situation. [21]

Chapter 6 Top Nine High Risk Incidents

A sample of types of incidents that result in a high risk of liability is explained below. The nine high risk events described below are based on statistics of sentinel (untoward) events kept by Joint Commission, the major accrediting body in the United States. They are also selected, based on my experience as a legal nurse consultant, in identifying the types of allegations that are difficult to defend.

The top nine high risk incidents are wrong site surgery, suicide, medication errors, delay in treatment, dropped while being transferred or anesthetized, sexual assault by employee or patient, retained surgical sponge or foreign object, and unnoticed cardiac arrest due to turning off alarms.

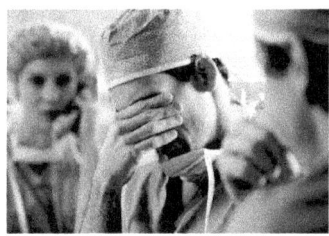

1. Wrong Site Surgery
Wrong site surgery means surgical procedures performed on the:

- wrong patient,
- wrong body part,
- wrong side or
- wrong level of a correctly identified anatomical site.

Types of surgeries that are at high risk for this error include, in descending order of frequency:

- orthopaedic surgery
- general surgery,
- neurosurgery,
- urologic surgery,

- dental/oral maxillofacial,
- cardiovascular-thoracic,
- ear-nose-throat, and
- ophthalmologic surgery.

Wrong site surgery occurs most often in an ambulatory surgery setting. Fifty-eight percent of the cases reported to Joint Commission occurred in either a hospital-based ambulatory surgery unit or freestanding ambulatory setting, with 29 percent occurring in the inpatient operating room and 13 percent in other inpatient sites such as the Emergency Department or ICU.

Seventy-six percent of wrong site surgery involved surgery on the wrong body part or site; 13 percent involved surgery on the wrong patient; and 11 percent involved the wrong surgical procedure. [22]

Risk Factors and Root Causes
The Joint Commission identified a number of factors contributing to the increased risk for wrong site, wrong person, or wrong procedure surgery, including:

- Emergency cases (19 percent).
- Unusual physical characteristics, including morbid obesity or physical deformity (16 percent).
- Unusual time pressures to start or complete the procedure (13 percent).
- Unusual equipment or set-up in the operating room (13 percent).
- Multiple surgeons involved in the case (13 percent).
- Multiple procedures being performed during a single surgical visit (10 percent).

The discovery process of a lawsuit often reveals the root causes associated with the chain of events that led to patient injury. The root causes identified by the operating room staff usually involved more than one factor; however, the majority involved a breakdown in communication between surgical team members and the patient and family. Other contributing causes included:

- Policy issues such as marking of the surgical site were not required.
- Verification in the operating room and a verification checklist were not required.
- Patient assessment was incomplete, including an incomplete pre-operative assessment.
- Staffing issues, distraction factors, availability of pertinent information in the operating room, and organizational cultural issues were also cited as contributing risk factors.

Risk reduction strategies are essential to assure the correct surgical site, patient and procedure by:

- Marking the surgical site and involving the patient in the marking process.
- Creating and using a verification checklist including appropriate documents, for example: medical records, X-rays and/or imaging studies.
- Obtaining oral verification of the patient, surgical site, and procedure in the operating room by each member of the surgical team.
- Monitoring compliance with these procedures.

Surgical teams, including the nursing staff, are required to take a "time out" in the operating room to verify the correct patient, procedure and site, using active (not passive) communication techniques. [23]

Case Example

While it is tempting to think of wrong site surgery as an issue that primarily affects operating room nurses, wrong site surgery could occur anywhere in the hospital where invasive procedures are performed. In a case that made headlines in November 2007, a neurosurgical resident began making an incision on the wrong side of the patient's head in an Intensive Care Unit. A travel nurse assisting him was unfamiliar with the hospital's policies requiring site verification. The patient, an 82-year-old woman, had bleeding between her brain and skull. The chief neurosurgery resident started to cut into the patient's head to remove the blood, but on the wrong side. The resident broke the skin but did not reach the skull. At that point the resident — a doctor in the seventh year of specialty training — realized the error and stopped the procedure.

The patient received one stitch to close the wound, and the procedure was then performed on the correct side, with good results. An investigation determined that no staff member who was present during the procedure had verified the surgical site as required by hospital policy. The Health Department's statement of deficiencies noted that "the nurse was a travel nurse and not familiar with the procedure." Every hospital which uses travel nurses must have procedures in place to make sure any newcomer knows the protocols. [24]

Case Example

In *Haile v. Sutherland*, 598 N.W. 2d 424 (Minn, 1999), the plaintiff was scheduled for the removal of a left axillary mass and a left chest lipomatous mass. After the surgery, it was discovered that the surgeon had instead removed benign tissue from her left breast. The surgeon claimed that the incorrect surgery was undertaken because the nurses had improperly draped the surgical site. After a series of legal maneuvers the case was resolved, but the court did not address the issue of improper draping. [25]

Feedback Question

What are the nurse's responsibilities related to incorrect surgery?

Answer

Nursing Responsibilities:

- Review the risk factors and root causes defined above to see how they apply.
- Be aware of the high risk situations to heighten awareness of the risks.
- Periodically participate in auditing the correct site verification forms and processes to ensure they are being accurately completed.
- Act as a preceptor for new personnel to inform them of the policy/procedure for site verification.
- Participate in correct site and patient identification as defined to include: the pre-procedure verification process, marking of the procedural site, performance of a time out before starting a procedure and assuring compliance with site verification procedures in non-traditional surgical areas for example, radiology suites, ambulatory clinics, and patient bedside. (Go to www.icsi.org for this paper – first edition 2006)

- Follow site verification policies which meet unique problems which have been identified through analysis of processes, systems and data.
- When surgery begins at change of shift, confirm that the previous shift has performed the site identification.
- Implement safety standard protocols for site verification.
- Do not allow surgeons, anesthesiologists or others to rush the site identification process.
- Follow the facility policy for patient disclosure for unanticipated outcomes. [26]

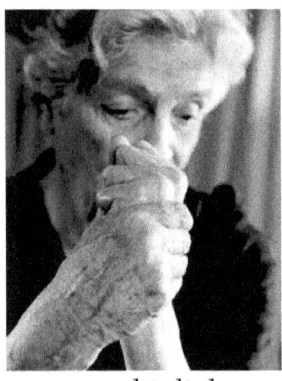

2. Suicide

Inpatient suicide is one of the most commonly reported sentinel events. (Reporting is voluntary and represents only a small number of actual events.) A patient can commit suicide anywhere in a hospital; this is not an issue confined to a psychiatric unit or hospital. Get updated statistics about sentinel events at this link:
http://www.jointcommission.org/Sentinel_Event_Trends_Reported_by_Year/

Feedback Question
Where do you think most suicides occur?
_Psychiatric hospital
_General hospital

Answer
If you picked psychiatric hospital, you are correct. A Joint Commission study of 65 cases of suicide revealed that most

of the suicides occurred in psychiatric hospitals, followed by general hospitals. Of the cases that occurred in general hospitals, 14 occurred in psychiatric units and 12 in medical surgical units. One occurred in the ER. In 75% of the cases, the method of suicide was a hanging in a bathroom, bedroom, or closet. Twenty percent of the suicides resulted from patients jumping from the roof or window. [27] A study of 22 fatal falls in 24-hour care settings showed that one third of the total falls were from what an expert called "extraordinary situations." These involved falling down a staircase or laundry chute or from an upper story window, roof or balcony. Seventeen of the 22 individuals had an altered mental status due to chronic mental illness or acute intoxication. [28]

Risk Factors

Telehealth nurses may receive calls from patients who are suicidal. Nurses should be alert to the risk factors and signs of suicidal intent. Risk factors include being unemployed, unmarried, having a problem with substance abuse, having a mood disorder, and a history of previous suicide attempts. Other risk factors include: a change in personality such as sad, withdrawn, irritable, anxious, tired, indecisive, or apathetic. There may be a change in behavior such as an inability to concentrate on school, work, or routine tasks or a change in sleep patterns characterized by oversleeping, insomnia, or early waking. Additional symptoms include a change in eating habits, loss of interest in people and activities previously enjoyed.

Suicidal patients may be worried about money or illness (real or imagined), feel like they are losing control, going crazy, or want to harm themselves or others, or have feelings of overwhelming guilt, shame, self-hatred. They may have no hope for the future or experienced a recent loss of relationship, marriage, house, job, or money. They may have nightmares and express suicidal impulses, or make statements, or plans. A classic warning sign is giving away favorite things. The suicidal patient may be agitated, hyperactive or restless.

Root Causes of Suicide
Studies of suicides show that several factors contributed to the heightened risk. These include:

- The environment of care, such as the presence of non-breakaway bars, rods or safety rails; lack of testing of breakaway hardware; and inadequate security.
- Patient assessment methods, such as incomplete suicide risk assessment at intake, absent or incomplete reassessment, and incomplete examination of the individual (for example, failure to identify a contraband).
- Staff-related factors, such as insufficient orientation or training, incomplete competency review or credentialing, and inadequate staffing levels.
- Incomplete or infrequent patient observations.
- Information-related factors such as incomplete communication among caregivers and information being unavailable when needed.
- Care planning, such as assignment of the patient to an inappropriate unit or location.

Case Example
In a Minnesota case, the plaintiff's decedent had a history of suicide attempts and had attempted to commit suicide on three occasions within three days shortly before confinement at the defendant's facility. The plaintiffs alleged that the facility failed to place the decedent in a closed or locked unit. The facility claimed that the decedent had to walk directly

past the nurse's station to escape from the facility. The plaintiff claimed that fifteen minute checks were ordered by the treating physician, but were not followed by staff. The plaintiff also claimed that the facility's staff observed the decedent leave the facility by cab. The decedent was later discovered in the backyard of the family home by his eldest son, having suffered a self-inflicted gunshot wound to the head. The plaintiff alleged negligence in the failure to supervise, watch and control the decedent. A $115,000 mediated settlement was reached. [29]

Case Example

In a Maryland case, an eighty-four year-old woman was admitted to the hospital for delirium and general IV hydration. Sometime in the evening hours, she was found dead on the ground outside her fourth floor hospital room. It was believed she had fallen through an open window in an attempt to leave the hospital. The plaintiffs alleged negligence in the failure to provide close observation in the form of a sitter or a bed alarm. The plaintiff also claimed that the hospital had no policy for keeping the windows locked and that there was no system in place for maintaining the key to relock the windows. The hospital admitted that there was no system in place for maintaining the key to relock the windows. A $430,000 jury verdict was returned. [30]

Physician Responsibilities

- A physician may be held liable if a patient commits suicide within a facility or shortly after discharge.
- The sooner the suicide occurs after discharge, the higher the liability.
- The physician may be liable if the patient should have been admitted to a facility and instead commits suicide.

- The physician's liability centers around control or prevention. It is more difficult to control the actions of an outpatient in the community than that of an inpatient who can be monitored, on one-to-one precautions, medicated, or restrained.
- Foreseeability is critical to a case where negligence is asserted involving a suicidal patient. The documentation should include:
  - An assessment of the patient's suicidal risk.
  - Information that alerts the clinician to the suicidal risk.
  - Knowledge of risk factors present including the patient's background.
  - Whether there were other low risk factors.
  - The questions posed by the clinician and the answers given by the patient.
  - How the information led to the actions taken. [31]

Feedback question
What should nurse managers do to reduce the risk of a suicide occurring in the clinical area?

Answer
Nurse manager responsibilities:
- Make a safety inspection of windows and bars in the rooms or request the assistance of the facility's safety committee to do so.
- Review the facility's admission assessment to determine what, if any, questions are routinely asked at the time of admission about suicidal thoughts.
- Review the orientation program to determine if information about suicide assessment is covered.

- Determine if sufficient staff are assigned to the unit to provide one to one monitoring, if such a practice is routinely provided on the unit.
- Audit charts of patients who are on one-to-one observations to determine if procedures are being followed. Make observations on the unit to spot check the compliance.
- Review the information being passed on about patients to determine if appropriate clinical data is being shared.
- Look at where a suicidal patient is being placed - at the end of a hall out of sight of the staff, or within vision?

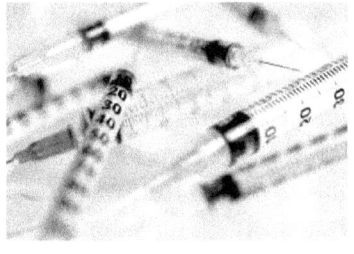

3. Injurious Medication Error
What are the five rights?
- Right drug
- Right route
- Right time
- Right patient
- Right dose

Most errors occur in the prescribing stage, followed by the administration stage. These situations require hypervigilance to avoid medication errors: drug dosing requires calculation, the patient is receiving IV medications, the patient needs several medications, the drug orders are handwritten, the patient is an infant, child or older adult, or the patient's health status is poor or critical.

The issue of high risk drugs has been extensively studied by the US Pharmacopoeia, and published in the form of a Med Marx report, the Institute for Safe Medication Practices, the

Institute for Healthcare Improvement, and the Joint Commission, among other agencies.

Several categories of high risk medications have been identified. Refer to the Institute for Safe Medication Practices (www.ismp.org) for a detailed list. [32] The highest risk medications include:

- Opiates (narcotics)
- Insulin
- Anticoagulants
- Anesthetics
- Sedatives
- Chemotherapeutic agents
- Neuromuscular blocking agents (cause respiratory paralysis)

The FDA released the results of an eight year study in the September 10, 2007 issue of Archives of Internal Medicine. [33] A study of adverse drug events that occurred from 1998 to 2005 showed that these events increased 2.6 fold from 35,000 to 90,000. Adverse drug events included adverse drug reactions, medication errors, accidental and intentional overdoses, and product problems. Three of the four drugs that caused the most deaths were opiates: Oxycodone, Fentanyl, and Morphine. The drugs causing the most disability were estrogens and insulin.

These factors contribute to medication errors:

- lack of knowledge,
- distractions,
- failure to follow the policies and procedures,
- failure to monitor,
- similar drug names, and

- packaging mix-ups

Case Example
The twenty-one year-old plaintiff went to an emergency room with nausea after taking too much Tylenol during her menstrual cycle. A nurse administered acetylcystine intravenously. The emergency room physician had never given the IV form of the drug to anyone before and the pharmacy there had never dispensed the drug. The pharmacist's prescription said that the drug, which is given in three stages, should run "times" four hours during the second date and "times" sixteen hours during the final stage. The prescription should have said that a single dose of the drug was to be over a certain period of time. The emergency room physician signed and entered the order written by the pharmacist without checking it. The nurse who began administering the drug had never given it before.

The result was a four times overdose during the second stage and a sixteen times overdose during the final stage of transfusion. The patient suffered seizures and a brain herniation. A $15.5 million settlement was reached. [34]

Feedback Question
What are the nursing responsibilities associated with giving an unfamiliar drug?

Answer
The nurse expected to review the administration guidelines and seek clarification from the pharmacist and drug literature. Ambulatory care nurses should be familiar with the medications they give and the expected side effects.

Case Example

The twenty-eight year-old plaintiff received the influenza vaccine from her family physician. Within 30 minutes, the plaintiff lost consciousness while driving. This caused her to lose control of her car. She suffered severe injuries and was hospitalized for 6 weeks. Her expert witness maintained she had a vasovagal reaction to the vaccine, which was not uncommon and was a universally recognized potential complication. The case settled for $246,415. [35]

The above case refers to a vaccine that was given. Another vaccine-related case focused on the failure to provide annual or preventive care to a patient.

Case Example

The plaintiff underwent a splenectomy in 1985. After the procedure, she received a pneumovas vaccination. She did not receive a hemophillus or meningococcal vaccination. In April 2001, at the age of thirty-five, she began seeing a new primary care physician. She saw the physician twice and a nurse practitioner four times. The plaintiff developed a pneumococcal infection that led to a three-month hospitalization. She became septic, had organ failure and necrosis and partial amputation of her toes. The plaintiff can walk only short distances now and suffers from chronic infection and pain. She claimed she should have been revaccinated for pneumococcal disease.

The defendants claimed the plaintiff's visits had all been for acute sick visits, not annual preventative and wellness physicals, which did not provide them an opportunity to recommend or administer a pneumococcal vaccine. The defendants also claimed that the pneumococcal vaccination is not the standard of care, has not been proven to be effective, and would not necessarily have prevented the plaintiff's infection. A $3 million settlement was reached. [36]

How Errors are Categorized

The Medication Error Council developed an index for categorizing errors. Their system is as follows:

Type of Error/Category	Result
No error	
Category A	Circumstances or events that have the capacity to cause error (this is the dangerous situation)
Error, No Harm	
Category B	An error occurred but the medication did not reach the patient
Category C	An error occurred that reached the patient but did not cause patient harm
Category D	An error occurred that resulted in the need for increased patient monitoring but no patient harm
Error, Harm	
Category E	An error occurred that resulted in the need for treatment or intervention and caused temporary patient harm
Category F	An error occurred that caused initial or prolonged hospitalization and caused temporary patient harm
Category G	An error occurred that resulted impermanent patient harm
Category H	An error occurred that resulted in a near-death event (e.g. anaphylaxis, cardiac arrest)
Error, Death	
Category I	An error occurred that resulted in patient death. [37]

Feedback Question
Identify actions that nurse managers can perform to reduce medication errors.

Answer
Nurse Manager Responsibilities:

- Identify the high risk medications routinely given in the employment setting.
- Make an inspection of medication administration areas for potential hazards.
- Emphasize the "no interruption rule" when nurses are preparing medications.
- Validate the medication administration skills of new hires with a checklist, if such a procedure is not in place.
- Be alert to look-alike sound-alike medications and post warning posters in the employment setting.
- Encourage the staff to educate patients and families about medications and teach them the importance of responding to any questioning by patients, particularly questions about new medications or routines.
- Work towards the implementation of bar code scanning for medication administration - a system that has been proven to reduce errors. If bar code scanning is in use, observe for any work arounds the system and if noted, reinforce proper use of the system.
- If intrathecal chemotherapy is administered on the nursing unit, do not permit intravenous medications to be administered at the same time in the same room. Many errors involving intrathecal medication administration involve inadvertent injection of drugs meant to be given by the intravenous route.

- Ensure staff members are aware of the hazards of PCA (patient controlled analgesia) by proxy, or permitting a family member or nurse to push the PCA button instead of the patient.
- Work with the physician staff to develop a standardized order sheet for PCA use and for administration of Heparin.
- Encourage staff to report near misses or hazardous situations that contribute to medication errors.
- Support a non-punitive environment so that staff who report medication errors are not punished for their actions, but rather encouraged to come forward.

Nursing Responsibilities Following a Medication Error

The standard of care requires that the nurse does the following after an error:

1. Report the error by notifying the nurse manager and the physician, who is ultimately responsible for determining how to treat the patient.
2. Make a baseline assessment to identify adverse reactions and evaluate response to any treatment.
3. If the organization has a risk manager, that individual may be involved in informing the patient about the error. In other settings, the physician will assume this responsibility. This is decided on a case-by-case basis.
4. File an incident report documenting the error so that corrective actions can be taken. Incident reports also alert the risk manager to trends or patterns. The report should describe the medication error accurately and concisely. For example, "Sinequan 25 mg ordered at 2000 but given at 0800 inadvertently." The

incident report is not supposed to offer excuses, such as "I was distracted and made an error."

5. The incident report may contain relevant information, such as a misplaced decimal point on the order form or a mislabeled medication container.

6. Report the error to the US Pharmacopeia or the Food and Drug Administration's MEDWATCH program.

7. Document and record any adverse reactions the patient suffered, and how the patient reacted when told about the error.

8. Document on the medical record. This step varies among institutions. Nurses are taught that if they are documenting the error somewhere else besides the incident report, not to use the word "error." [38]

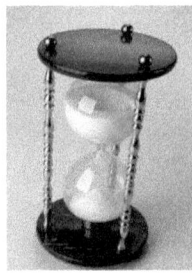

4. Delay in Treatment

A delay in treatment can close a window of opportunity to change the outcome- such as in spinal cord compression, compartment syndrome, fetal distress, bowel evisceration, rupturing aortic aneurysm, respiratory distress, hemorrhage, and other conditions.

Nurses are expected to act as patient advocates to secure help for their patients. Failure to rescue describes clinicians' inability to save a patient's life when he experiences a complication.

Case Example
The plaintiff's decedent, age twenty-one months, became ill in late January 2008, with a low grade fever, vomiting, and unwillingness to stand or walk. The pediatrician was called and influenza was initially diagnosed during a conversation with a nurse. Three days later a diagnosis of gastroenteritis was made following an office examination of the child, which lasted less than ten minutes. The child cried louder than his father ever heard him cry during the abdominal exam, but the pediatrician told the father that his appendix was fine.

No laboratory or imaging studies were done in connection with the exam. The child died at home the next day. It was determined that the child had a gangrenous appendix which had leaked bacteria into his abdomen. Autopsy findings were that the acute abdominal process had been present for 48-120 hours prior to death. The case went to jury and resulted in an award of $1,267,234.02. [39]

Feedback Question
Was the office nurse negligent?

Answer
The nurse's responsibility was to gather information but not make a medical diagnosis. There is not enough information in the above case description about how the nurse arrived at the diagnosis of influenza, if indeed it was the nurse's diagnosis.

Staffing and Staff Mix
The quality of nursing care is directly affected by staffing and hiring decisions.

What do we know about staffing and delays in treatment or patient safety issues? Most of the research investigated staffing in hospitals.

- Nurses are better able to detect changes in condition that warrant intervention when the nurse-patient ratio is low and there are a greater proportion of registered nurses on the staff.
- Higher nurse-to-patient ratios are associated with improved patient outcomes, affecting both morbidity (illness) and mortality (death).
- An American Nurses Association study [40] found that higher nurse-to-patient ratios were associated with shorter lengths of stay in hospitals and a reduction in complications such as pressure sores, pneumonia, urinary tract and postoperative infections.
- A California study showed that impact on patient outcomes and registered nurse skill mix. There was an association between total nursing hours per patient and two outcomes: urinary tract infections and length of stay. A stronger association was observed between the registered nurse proportions of the total nursing hours of care and the same outcomes. The higher the total nursing hours per patient day and registered nurse proportion, the lower the length of stay and the lower the odds of hospitalized patients developing urinary tract infections. [41]
- A large-scale study of 589 randomly selected community hospitals [42] found an inverse relationship between the number of registered nurses and adverse events following surgery. In other words, the fewer the registered nurses, the more frequent the complications.

- The largest of studies on nurse staffing (jointly funded by AHRQ, the Health Resources and Services Administration, the Centers for Medicare and Medicaid Services, and the National Institute of Nursing Research) [43] examined the records of 5 million medical patients and 1.1 million surgical patients who had been treated at 799 hospitals during 1993. Among the study's principal findings were:
  - Hospitals with high registered nurse staffing had medical patients with lower rates of urinary tract infections, pneumonia, shock, upper gastrointestinal bleeding, and shorter hospital stays than patients in hospitals with low registered nurse staffing.
  - Major surgery patients in hospitals that were better staffed had lower rates of urinary tract infections and failure to rescue (failure to intervene to address a complication).
  - Higher rates of registered nurse staffing were associated with a 3 to 12 percent reduction in adverse outcomes.
  - Higher staffing at all levels of nursing was associated with a 2 to 25 percent reduction in adverse outcomes.

The hours of staffing difference were significant in this study. The hospitals with higher hours of registered nurse staffing (75th percentile) had an average of 9.1 hours of inpatient RN nursing per patient day, while those with lower RN staffing (25th percentile) had an average of 6.4 hours of inpatient RN nursing per patient day. Hospitals with a higher percentage of RN staffing (75th percentile) had an average of 75 percent of inpatient nursing hours provided by RNs. Those with lower RN staffing (25th percentile) had an average of 63 percent of nursing hours provided by RNs.

More nurses at the bedside could save thousands of patient lives each year.

- Every additional patient in an average hospital nurse's workload increased the risk of death in surgical patients by 7 percent.
- Patients with life-threatening complications were also less likely to be rescued in hospitals where nurses' patient loads were heavier.
- Costs may increase when there are too few nurses due to the high costs of replacing burnt-out nurses and higher costs of caring for patients with poor outcomes.
- A study examined data collected from 168 hospitals, 232,342 surgical patients, and 10,184 nurses in Pennsylvania from 1998 to 1999. The researchers examined data from relatively common general surgeries (such as gall bladder removal), orthopaedic surgery (knee or hip replacement), and vascular surgeries excluding cardiac surgery such as coronary bypass.) [44] The findings of this study were confirmed by examination of 26 studies, most of which examined nurse staffing levels and adverse occurrences in the hospital setting, including in-hospital deaths and nonfatal adverse outcomes such as nosocomial (hospital-acquired) infections, pressure ulcers or falls. Lower nurse to patient ratios were associated with higher rates of nonfatal adverse outcomes.

Staffing and the Telehealth Nurse
Ideally, the nurse answering calls from patients is assigned only to that function. Distraction and time pressure can cause the nurse to not recognize the significance of a finding, overlook questions to be asked, or lose track of the information being shared.

Critical Thinking Errors

The telehealth nurse is expected to use critical thinking to evaluate the patient. Facilities may provide and use clinical support tools to guide the telehealth nurse's practice. They fortify but do not replace the use of the nursing process and clinical critical thinking. Protocols are useful for giving guidance in situations, but cannot predict the unusual circumstance that demands critical thinking. The expression "rules are meant to be broken" may have applicability in those situations when the nurse must act as a patient advocate to gain attention for the patient.

Overconfidence

Just as too little experience can result in errors, too much confidence in one's own abilities and experience can increase the likelihood of error. Overconfidence can result in incorrect use of the nursing process. For example, the overconfident nurse may not perform an adequate assessment by failing to gather enough information the patient's status. Factors that contribute to overconfidence include:

1. Large amounts of positive feedback from peers, other professionals, or the public
2. The reliance on unaided memory
3. The lack of awareness of environmental or treatment effects on outcomes (i.e., focusing on outcome feedback as opposed to process feedback)
4. The failure to search for disconfirming evidence
5. Enjoying a feeling of control and self-confidence

Components of overconfidence include:

1. The failure to consider alternative perspectives
2. The failure to distinguish inferences from assertions

3. Favoring positive over negative information
4. Unwarranted certainty in the individual's accuracy of prediction

Case Example

I reviewed a case as an expert witness that involved a patient who was to have surgery for glaucoma. The same day surgery nurse was being sued for medications she gave the patient. This nurse was confident she knew what preoperative medications were required. Further, she thought the physician forgot to provide preoperative eye drop orders. The nurse created an order sheet listing the medications she thought the doctor would order, and wrote up the orders as a telephone order from the eye surgeon, although she did not speak to the surgeon. The nurse administered the eye drops to the patient. Unfortunately, the medications the nurse administered were contraindicated for the type of glaucoma the patient had.

The surgeon tried to reverse the effects of the medications the preop nurse gave, and went ahead with the surgery. The patient had a poor outcome and lost vision. The case was settled; the physician's and nurse's insurance companies paid the claim.

Bias

Assigning labels to patients can cause the nurse to skip an adequate assessment. Think of the nurses who see the same patients over and over and develop an opinion that the person is malingering, seeking attention, too anxious, or drug seeking. Creating stereotypes based on culture, age, or frequency of contact with the ambulatory care nurse can lead to oversights in assessment.

Risk of Errors Based on Lack of Knowledge

The measurement criteria of Standard 1 of the AAACN standards states that telehealth nurses are professional licensed registered nurses with appropriate education and work experience. The standard also addresses the need for written job descriptions that define the responsibilities and performance measurements of telehealth nursing staff.

Can a clerical person safely gather the information to route the call to the right person? Is having a list of red flat symptoms safe? What happens if the patient says she is having severe indigestion? Or jaw pain? Or a very bad headache? Should clerical people do first level triage? What is the risk? (This person's inability to recognize key findings, the nature and urgency of the call can be underestimated, resulting in a delay in care.)

Lack of Visual Information: What You Can't See Can Hurt the Patient

How much of our communication is visual versus verbal? Think about how we rely on facial expressions and nonverbal language. How much information can we gather over the phone? The telehealth nurse cannot confirm information by looking at the patient. You should err on the side of caution. The patient may say, "I am concerned. I want to be seen. Something is not right". A rule of thumb is if the nurse (or the patient) is concerned, the patient should probably be seen promptly. The adage is, "If in doubt, send them out".

Accepting the Patient's Diagnosis

Not taking the time to investigate abnormal findings as reported by ancillary staff or other nurses may result in injury. Patients may be right about what is wrong with them, but they can also be very wrong. The nurse has to use his or her education to perform critical thinking to delve into the symptoms.

Not Functioning Within Job Description
In the following case, the physician used an unlicensed person to perform tasks that more clearly belonged to the role of a registered nurse.

Case Example
The plaintiff, age forty-two, had a ten-year history of Type 2 diabetes when he went to the emergency room with a groin boil and fever. The defendant emergency room physician lanced the boil and prescribed antibiotics, but did not order any culture studies or lab studies before instructing the plaintiff to follow up at the local clinic. Four days later, the plaintiff had an ongoing fever and another groin boil. Over the next several days, the plaintiff returned to the clinic and the emergency department where he was seen by the defendant due to persistent fever, lethargy, and ongoing infection. The infection was now spreading from the groin to the buttocks, abdomen and low back.

The plaintiff was eventually seen by a different physician in the emergency room, who correctly diagnosed Fournier's Gangrene. The plaintiff was stabilized and transferred to another hospital, where he was treated for sepsis and aggressive debridements of dead tissue throughout the perineum and abdominal area. The plaintiff learned through the lawsuit that the physician was uninsured. The doctor had a history of malpractice claims and multiple instances of board discipline. At the doctor's deposition, he admitted permitting his bookkeeper, who had no formal medical training or license to provide medical care, assess the plaintiff and inject antibiotics when he was not at the clinic. The case settled for $925,000. [45]

The next case highlights the limitations of the medical assistant role.

Intimidation Affects Delays in Treatment

Nurses who detect signs of a potentially serious complication must mobilize resources quickly, including the ability to bring the patient into the office for evaluation. Intimidation may play a role in preventing nurses from quickly reacting to a change in the patient's condition. The telehealth nurse may be reluctant to be perceived as overreacting. Nurses who are fearful of being criticized for erring on the side of caution may hold back from giving the patient direction to be seen to be evaluated. This advice to be evaluated may be in the patient's best interest.

Nurses are team players. Nurses are expected to collaborate with others. A telephone triage nurse may err by not doing something he or she should, such as asking the patient to come to the doctor's office, or go to the emergency department. On the other hand, the nurse's decision making may be questioned if the urgent appointment turns out to be unnecessary. One of the ways to combat this is to discuss the risks of each course and make it an explicit part of the culture to state that the triage nurse can never be wrong if she refers the patient to be seen.

Failure to consider all of the available information can result in mistaken diagnoses. Both nurses and physicians are prone to this trap. This may result from rushing through a call in order to reach a conclusion.

Case Example

This obstetrics example is a perfect illustration of the results of intimidation. In *Anonymous Parents and Deceased Five-year-Old Girl v. Anonymous Obstetrician and Anonymous Hospital*, the plaintiffs alleged their infant developed cerebral palsy after a difficult labor and delivery. Deposition testimony of the labor and delivery nurses indicated they were concerned about the lack of progress of the mother's labor, but they were reluctant to voice those concerns to the obstetrician because of the doctor's well-known tendency to respond negatively to such nursing input. This North Carolina case settled for $1.2 million. [46]

Bullying

A study of 2,095 healthcare providers revealed that intimidating behaviors are far from isolated events. In one year, 88% had encountered condescending language or voice intonation; 87% encountered impatience with questions, and 79% encountered reluctance or refusal to answer questions or return phone calls. Sixty nine percent reported that physician/prescribers had often (12%) or at some time during the past year (57%) stated: "Just give what I ordered." Consequently, 49% of the respondents said that intimidation had altered the way they handled order clarification or questions about medication orders. At least once during the past year, about 40% of the respondents who had concerns about a medication order assumed it was correct, or asked another professional to talk to the prescriber, rather than interact with the intimidating prescriber. Another large group of respondents (75%) sought the help of colleagues to help interpret an order rather than contact the prescriber. Seven percent of the respondents had been involved in a medication error in which intimidation clearly played a role. [47]

Sometimes failure to rescue occurs because of intimidation. This is developing into a hot topic in nursing as individuals recognize that miscommunication can occur because that healthcare provider is very difficult to approach, whether that's another nurse, a person of the same background or at a different level.

Horizontal or lateral violence is the term that refers to workplace hostility. It's not confined to healthcare settings. It's a problem in the corporate world as well and other work places where there's aggression or hostility or criticism coming either from a person from that same level or from a different level.

The impact on nursing has been studied. It's been found that 60% of newly registered nurses leave their job in the first year due to some form of horizontal violence. We spend all this money training individuals, then we lose them because of a hostile atmosphere. Bullying exacts a huge personal and financial cost. The way to combat this is assertiveness skills, teaching people how to confront, and how to communicate better.

Firmer steps are being taken to impose a zero tolerance policy for abusive behavior as the negative effects of disruptive behavior are recognized. In some VHA hospitals, the physicians sign a conduct contract. The first instance of abusive behavior is treated with counseling. The second incident results in termination. Physicians <u>are</u> being fired. [48] Joint Commission standards address the need to identify disruptive behavior and to change the culture so it is not permitted.

Feedback Question
What are nursing responsibilities to avoid delays in treatment?

Answer
- Recognize your role as a patient advocate.

- It is imperative that telehealth nurses detect signs of a critical change in patient's condition and intervene as early as possible.
- Although unlicensed, assistive personnel may collect data. It is up to the registered nurse to review the data to look for trends in a patient's condition. It is up to the registered nurse answering calls through telephone triage to recognize the serious symptoms that warrant timely evaluation.
- Inexperienced staff nurses should seek guidance from more experienced staff members.
- Staff nurses must be persistent in carrying concerns up the chain of command until resolution of concerns has occurred.

Feedback Question
What can nurse managers do to reduce delays in treatment from occurring?

Answer
Nurse Manager Responsibilities:
- Work with administration to secure adequate staffing. Recognize that skill mix and experience are important. Avoid staffing with a group of inexperienced nurses.
- Discuss the chain of command with the staff - when and how it should be used. Impress upon the staff that it will be difficult to defend a nurse who did not speak up when a clinical problem was evident because it might affect the relationship with the physician, or the physician did not do anything with the concerning information. The nurse must consult with the nurse manager to go up the chain of command to secure help for the patient.

- Work with administration to develop a zero tolerance of abusive behavior by staff.

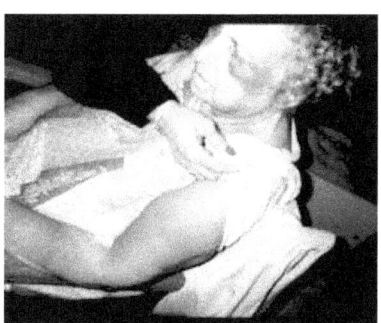

5. Dropped During Transfer or While Anesthetized
Nursing staff are expected, according to the standard of care, to use the appropriate number of staff and equipment needed to safely move a patient. A drop during transfer may result in fractured extremities, spinal cord injury, head trauma, and soft tissue injuries. Damages are compounded if the patient is receiving anticoagulation in the form of Heparin, Coumadin, Lovenox and other anticoagulants.

A drop during transfer can occur under the following circumstances:

The nurse rolls the patient over in bed without putting up the side rail. The patient falls off the bed or is rolled off a stretcher. These types of incidents are rare. The following types of situations are more common:

- The patient is dropped from a Hoyer lift because of failure to control the equipment or attempting to handle the lift without adequate help.
- The patient is dropped during a transfer from a bed or stretcher to a chair or chair to wheelchair or examining table.
- The Hoyer lift sling is improperly laundered and tears during use, dropping the patient on the floor.

Although this topic is devoted to drops during handling, there are lesser injuries that may occur during patient handling, such as injuries when a caregiver lifts or tugs at a patient's arms or lifts under her shoulders, or creates skin tears or bruises. These types of injuries are rarely the focus of litigation, as the damages do not justify the expense of litigation. However, the injuries may raise concern in family members about mistreatment or abuse.

The healthcare industry acknowledges that manual patient handling is not safe - either for the patient or for the nurse at risk for musculoskeletal injuries from lifting, transporting, and repositioning patients. Yet relatively few United States healthcare facilities have an adequate number of mechanical lifting and repositioning aids. Even when such aids are available, many nurses resist using them, despite evidence that manual handling causes injury. During a typical 8 hour shift, a nurse lifts a cumulative weight of about 1.8 tons. As most shifts are 12 hours, the lifting is even worse. As patients become heavier, patient handling becomes more burdensome. [49]

The patient may fall if caregivers neglect to assess her handling requirements and physical abilities. Delay in recognition of the injury worsens the problem. Instead of properly assessing the pain in terms of onset, associated symptoms, radiation, or ability to bear weight, the staff may medicate the patient with an analgesic. This may compound the original injury given the fact that a previous body movement (transitioning from bed to wheelchair with assistance) took place.

Falls may take place in the ambulatory care environment. They may occur when a patient is getting on or off an examining table, when recovering from anesthesia, after blood has been taken, and in other circumstances.

Case Example

The plaintiff, who was in her eighties, was at the office of her eye doctor for laser surgery. Her vision was poor in that she was not allowed to drive at night. After her pupils were dilated, she was brought to the laser room and told by an assistant to sit on a chair with rollers. The seat rolled out from under her as she attempted to sit. The plaintiff suffered a fractured ankle. She has an extended hospitalization. She claimed it was inappropriate to have a seat with rollers used by patients with poor vision. The case settled for $220,000.[50]

Concealment

I've seen several instances of lawsuits that resulted from falls associated with nursing assistants who got people out of bed with Hoyer lifts. Because of the sling not being correctly positioned or a patient movement or the balance being off, patients can fall out of lifts. Typically they fracture a hip or hit their heads. I've reviewed medical records of lawsuits in which the nursing assistants were afraid to tell anybody about the fall. They knew they'd get in trouble or lose their jobs. So they didn't say anything. There was no description of an incident. They did not tell the nurse on duty. The fractured hip was discovered later in that shift or the next day. The next nurse may observe the patient has an externally rotated leg, a shortened extremity, and is complaining of pain. An x-ray shows a fracture.

The individual or individuals involved in the incident may be fearful of reporting the injury, hoping that no one will become aware of the event. An incident that occurs during the transfer of a patient may not be documented by the staff involved. In the absence of documentation about an incident, the defense may argue that the fracture was pathological or spontaneous. Spontaneous fractures are fractures that occur without the degree of trauma that would generally be accepted as being necessary to break a bone. They are commonly associated with disease conditions that impair bone strength, such as cancer and Paget's disease.

There have been few reports of spontaneous fractures of the shafts of long bones. Two authors [51, 52] who studied this clinical issue found that pathological fractures were quite rare. Determining the cause of fractures is often difficult and debated amongst orthopaedic and endocrinology experts. Most traumatic fractures resulting from falls in the elderly involve fractures of the wrist or hip. Pathological fractures are most often due to osteoporosis, hypoparathyroidism or malignant metastases and are not often immediately recognized. In addition to fractures of long bones, pathological fractures may involve the vertebra.

Staff members are supposed to use care when handling the patient who is anesthetized. In the following case, a physician was injured while she was sedated for a colonoscopy.

Case Example
The plaintiff, a seventy-year-old pediatrician in active practice, presented to the defendants for a routine colonoscopy on July 23, 2003. During preparation for the procedure, she was sedated and the bed rail was lowered. While unobserved, the plaintiff fell from the bed and struck her head on the floor. Sedation was reversed and the plaintiff was transported to the hospital where she received stitches and was released. Upon returning home, the plaintiff continued to experience dizziness, disorientation, vomiting

and difficulty performing daily activities. She was admitted to a hospital and post-concussive syndrome was diagnosed. Thereafter, the plaintiff sought care at a university hospital where traumatic brain injury was diagnosed.

She will require monitoring by a neurologist and a psychiatrist for the rest of her life and is unable to live alone, drive a car or practice medicine. The defense denied that the plaintiff sustained a traumatic brain injury and claimed that she had pre-existing psychiatric problems. According to published accounts, the case settled for a confidential sum in mediation. [53]

Feedback Question
What are the responsibilities to reduce the incidence of patients being dropped or falling during handling?

Answer
Institutional Responsibilities:
- Work with the staff development department to ensure that periodic in-services are provided on safe patient handling techniques.
- Determine if the nursing administration has a committee reviewing ways to add more, if needed, patient handling aids. Many devices are on the market to assist in this effort, including lateral transfer aid, full body floor lifts, sit to stand lifts, standing assistance aids, overhead ceiling track systems, and slings.
- Ensure staff members are performing accurate fall risk assessments upon admission and thereafter according to policy.
- Work with administration to provide sufficient physical therapy resources to promote physical conditioning.

- Ask the safety committee, if one exists, to examine the patient care environment for assistive devices that improve mobility and safety, such as grab bars, hand rails, raised toilet seats, lockable wheelchairs, good lighting, low bed heights, bed alarms, floor mats, and other safety devices.
- Review the fall alert program to determine if it specifically advises staff and visitors of the patient's risk for falls.
- Ensure there is a comprehensive clinical and risk evaluation after a fall.
- Ensure that falls are tracked through the quality improvement program, and opportunities for improvement are identified and addressed.
- Obtain support of the administration for purchase of the required equipment, commitment of resources for staff training, and dissemination of policies which prohibit manual lifting.
- Discuss with the staff the importance of reporting incidents of patients being dropped so that adequate medical assessment can be performed.
- Help the staff realize that concealing an incident will worsen liability and increase the difficulty of defending a suit.

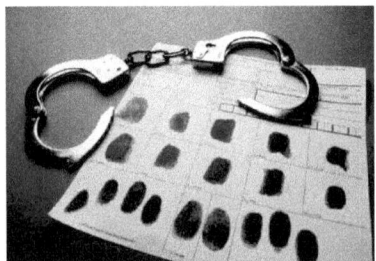

6. Sexual Assault by Employee or Patient
Sexual assault is a particularly heinous crime, and one that harms the patient, damages the reputation of the healthcare facility, and may lead to a lawsuit that is difficult to defend. In many states,

registered nurses are mandatory reporters, who must report actual or suspected neglect or abuse of a vulnerable adult (or child).

Healthcare administrators are charged with the responsibility to perform an investigation of a potential new hire to see if that individual has a criminal background. Additionally the facility's staff should determine if the employee ever worked for the facility before and if so, was he or she the object of any disciplinary action or termination.

Sexual assault may occur as a result of patient-to-patient contact, employee to patient contact, visitor to patient contact, or intruder to patient contact.

Signs of possible sexual abuse: [54] [55] [56]

- Rectal or genital bruising, bleeding or discharge.
- Genital, rectal, or urinary irritation, injury, infection, or scarring.
- Sexually transmitted diseases.
- Sperm in a female's urine.
- Torn, stained, or bloody underwear.
- Difficulty walking or sitting due to genital discomfort.
- Injuries in various stages of healing or that are not readily explained.
- Withdrawal, anxiety, depression, humiliation, embarrassment, guilt, self-blame, low self-esteem, hopelessness, helplessness.
- Bruises, restraint marks on wrists or ankles.
- Troubled sleep and disturbing dreams.
- Behavior changes when a certain person is around.
- Anxiety, exaggerated startle response, panic attacks.
- Anger.

- Bruises, abrasions, lacerations of the neck, trunk, or extremities.
- Rope burns of the wrist/ankle (where victim was tied down during assault).
- Exacerbation of underlying chronic illness such as hypertension and diabetes.
- Fatigue.

What are the Damages?

One of the defenses of sexual assault cases is to minimize the damages. However, research shows that post traumatic stress disorder is a prevalent problem after a sexual assault. Foa and Rothbaum [57] found that nearly 50% of women who are raped suffer from post traumatic stress disorder (PTSD). Adjustment disorder and acute stress disorder may follow. Fields [58] states that data on PTSD in the elderly suggest that age "contributes minimally" to the prediction of PTSD. Pre-existing physical and mental health, severity of the trauma, and specific resources have greater predictive potency. [59]

Case Example

A Maryland woman was suffering from Alzheimer's disease. She was allegedly raped by another nursing home resident, and additionally suffered physical assault on multiple occasions at the hands of other residents. After her sexual assault, she was taken to a hospital for a post-rape medical workup. She also suffered psychological injuries from her mental deficits. The plaintiff alleged that the nursing home violated its standard of care in failing to provide adequate security to protect the patient from other assaultive residents, and from herself. The defendant denied liability, but agreed to settle the case for $800,000. [60]

An interesting Hawaii case reveals issues related to supervision of employees assigned to patients.

Case Example

The plaintiff's wife, age twenty-five, was brought to the emergency room of Tripler Army Medical Center in March 2001 in a comatose state. She had collapsed in a club in Pearl Harbor Naval Station. The initial diagnosis was acute intoxication, primary seizure disorder, toxic ingestion (suspected date rape type drug), knee and head injuries and infection. She was transferred to the lCU and remained sedated/unconscious during the day. The night shift in the ICU included three registered nurses and a male LPN. The LPN was assigned to monitor the plaintiff's seizures and stay in her private room all night. The three other nurses were assigned to six other patients.

The charge nurse came into the plaintiff's room just before midnight and took a quick glance, noticing that the LPN was rubbing lotion on the plaintiff's legs and the plaintiff was sleeping or unconscious. The charge nurse next entered the plaintiff's room about four and one-half hours later. The plaintiff claimed that the LPN applied baby lotion four times (massages) during the shift and that during the third massage, which occurred just prior to the second visit by the charge nurse. He became sexually aroused and sexually assaulted the plaintiff (digitally penetrating her vagina). The LPN later pled guilty to a count of sexual assault, although he claimed the sexual acts were consensual. The plaintiff claimed that the incident caused pain due to the bumping of the catheter which was in place at the time. The plaintiff claimed that she tried to push the LPN away when he placed his mouth over her left breast, but did not have muscle control and could not call out. The plaintiff claimed that the ICU was understaffed, that the LPN was negligently supervised, the massage seen by the charge nurse during her first look should have alerted her to something unusual, the

ICU room door should have remained open, the hospital's chaperone policy was violated and the hospital was negligent in that the sexual assault was foreseeable.

The defendant argued that the lCU's capacity was eight and that with seven patients the staffing level was appropriate. The defendant also claimed that increased staffing, or use of a chaperone, would not have prevented the assault and that the observation by the charge nurse did not raise any concern because it was not unusual for a nurse to apply lotion to a patient who was not awake, both for circulatory purposes and skin care. The defendant also claimed that having the door closed was not negligent and that personnel other than the charge nurse were in the room at times.

The defendant also claimed that the LPN had no criminal history or history of professional misconduct and that allowing several hours to pass without direct supervision was not negligent. The defense also argued that the court did not have subject matter jurisdiction because of the limited waiver of immunity under the Federal Tort Claims Act. The court, however, found that the claims were not barred. The court also found that the hospital knew of the risk of assault on patients, citing the chaperone policy. According to Personal Injury Judgments Hawaii, a $906,000 award was given. This included $186,000 for the plaintiff and $90,000 for her husband. [61]

Feedback Question
What are the institutional responsibilities for addressing the potential problem of a sexual assault?

Answer
Institutional Responsibilities:

- Be aware if nursing staff are required by state law to report suspicions of abuse. If so, periodically reaffirm the responsibility of nursing staff to report these concerns. Mandatory reporting of concerns about abuse is required in nursing home settings.
- Ensure that screening of new hires investigates prior convictions of sexual assault.
- Encourage staff to take seriously any comment made by a patient about inappropriate sexual contact. Many people erroneously think that rape is a sexually motivated act rather than an act of violence.
- Promote education related to the facility's written policy against sexual abuse.
- Protect patients from abuse from other patients.
- Ensure staff is aware of the importance of preserving evidence, such as not bathing a patient who alleges a sexual assault, before an examination and rape kit test is done.

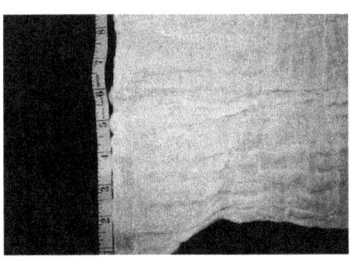

7. Retained Surgical Sponge or Foreign Object

A retained foreign object is the most common basis for a malpractice claim against the operating room staff. Objects routinely used in operations that may be improperly retained include needles, sponges, laparotomy pads, and medical instruments such as Kelly clamps, hemostats or scissors. Cases of this kind are usually brought under the *res ipsa loquitur* theory, or "the thing speaks for itself." In some states, the surgeon is held to be negligent when an incorrect count is performed; in other states, the surgeon is absolved of liability because of lack of direct involvement in the negligent act of counting the sponges or instruments after their use, unless the surgeon knew of the incorrect count and did nothing.

The purpose of the initial count is to establish a baseline accounting of all instruments, sharps, sponges and miscellaneous items prior to commencing a surgical procedure. Counts continue throughout the surgical procedure as items are added to the surgical field to replenish supplies such as laparotomy sponges, sutures and so on. Reflecting the collaborative atmosphere in the operating room, surgical counts are then performed:

- Before closure of a cavity within a cavity (e.g., a Caesarean would require an incision be made into the uterus).
- Before wound closure commences.
- At skin closure or end of the procedure.
- At a time of permanent relief assignment of either the scrub technician or the circulating nurse. [62]

Case Example

The twenty-five year-old plaintiff delivered a baby by cesarean section. During the procedure, a laparotomy pad was left inside her abdomen. She subsequently experienced abdominal pain, bleeding, and eventually diarrhea. The plaintiff was readmitted to the hospital 3 months later, at which time a CT scan revealed the lap pad. She had surgery to remove the pad and the abscess that formed around it. She was hospitalized for a week. She was also diagnosed with ulcerative colitis. The plaintiff contended that the retained lap pad caused or contributed to her ulcerative colitis and that she would require colon removal surgery in the future. The surgeon and the circulating nurse's employer/agency settled the case for $525,000. The hospital admitted liability several months prior to trial, but denied that the retained sponge caused the ulcerative colitis and claimed that the damages should be limited to the consequences stemming from the pad removal surgery.

The defendant claimed there is no known cause for ulcerative colitis. The jury returned a verdict of $1,367,500. The previous settlement was subtracted from this amount and the final figure was $842,500. [63]

Feedback Question

Earlier in this book you learned that a plaintiff has to prove the healthcare provider had a duty to the patient, the provider breached the duty, that there were damages, and that the breach in duty caused the damages. What aspect of these four elements was most strongly highlighted in the above case description?

Answer

This case focused heavily on the damages or the injuries to the patient that resulted from the retention of the lap pad.

Feedback Question

Which element was the basis of the defense?

Answer

The defense disputed the proximate cause between the breach in the standard of care (leaving a lap pad in) and the damages (ulcerative colitis).

Feedback Question

What can nurse managers do to reduce the risk of retained foreign objects?

Answer

Nurse Manager Responsibilities:

- Emphasize the importance of strictly following the procedures concerning surgical counts.
- Counting policies and procedures should be included in orientation as well as ongoing perioperative education to ensure skills development as well as enhancing attitudes which affect patient safety outcomes.
- Policies and procedures should be reviewed annually, revised as necessary and made readily available to all personnel in the practice setting
- Develop and implement a chain of command policy to ensure surgical counting and safety policy initiatives achieve safe patient outcomes.
- Encourage staff to act as patient advocates by invoking the chain of command and insisting on the investigation of inaccurate counts - before the patient leaves the operating room.
- As per facility policy, documentation of counts performed should be retained in the department records. Do spot audits of charts to determine if counts are being accurately recorded.

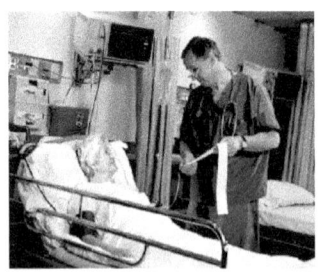

8. Unnoticed Cardiac or Respiratory Arrest due to Turning off the Alarms

Safety alarms exist to protect the patient from clinical problems. The maintenance of the alarms is of utmost importance as an early warning system.

There are several kinds of alarms in use in healthcare environments: on infusion pumps, cardiac monitors, ventilators, feeding pumps, doors and beds, among others.

Root cause analysis of 23 cases of ventilator-related deaths and injuries showed these alarm-related issues:

- The alarm was off or set incorrectly: 22%
- No alarm was present for certain disconnections of the ventilator: 22%
- The alarm was not audible in all areas: 22%
- The alarms were not tested: 13% [64]

Death and injury due to faulty alarms, inadequate alarm systems, alarm misuse, and airway disconnect are avoidable.

- The key is an informed and alert caregiver team.
- Staffing must be sufficient to provide professionals to hear the alarms. In a busy recovery room, alarms go off so frequently that nurses can become desensitized and may not race to the bedside every time an alarm sounds.
- The Joint Commission noted that 65 percent of recent sentinel events involving ventilator-related deaths were due to malfunction or misuse of an alarm, or an inadequate alarm.
- Critical care policy usually states that the patient alarms are never to be turned "off."
- Most monitoring systems or ventilators have the capacity to temporarily silence the alarm for approximately 15 seconds without terminating the system, or disconnecting the monitoring equipment. [65]

Feedback Question

What should the nurse manager do to reduce the risk of alarms being turned off and an arrest occurring?

Answer
Nurse Manager Responsibilities

- Professionals responsible for application, adjustment and monitoring of ventilators, alarm systems and airways, should possess relevant education, and have undergone validated competency testing.
- Systems are in place to check ventilator and monitoring system performance before and during clinical use.
- All devices and systems are maintained according to manufacturers' specification.
- A tracking system is in place to identify, analyze and remedy all ventilator-related incidents that lead to serious injury or death.
- Protocols for the application and discontinuance of mechanical ventilation are in place.
- A mechanism is in place to track outcomes of all ventilator patients.
- Organized, periodic, ventilator-related continuing education is accessible to those professionals responsible for the many components of care directed to ventilator patients.
- Establish new processes for alarm testing and verification of alarm settings.
- Establish new or redesigned alarm response procedures.
- Redesign rooms or units to improve observation of patient and ventilator.
- Improve and expand preventive maintenance on ventilators.
- Review orientation and training programs for job-specific, ventilator safety-related content and include in competency assessment process.

- Review staffing process to ensure effective staffing for ventilator patients at all times.
- Implement regular preventive maintenance and testing of alarm systems.
- Ensure that alarms are sufficiently audible with respect to distances and competing noise within the unit.
- Initiate interdisciplinary team training for staff caring for ventilator patients.
- Direct observation of ventilator-dependent patients is preferred in order to avoid over dependence on alarms. [66]

Case Example

The plaintiff's decedent, age forty-nine, was a patient at St. Barnabas Hospital's ICU. He was suffering from severe pancreatitis. He suffered cardiac arrest and died. The plaintiff claimed that a monitor beeped when his heart stopped, but his nurse had been called away to care for another patient. The alert did not show up on the nurses' central monitor because of faulty wiring. When a power outage caused a switch over to generator power, the monitor did not come back on. A settlement was reached for $1.2 million. The hospital and equipment manufacturer paid the award. [67]

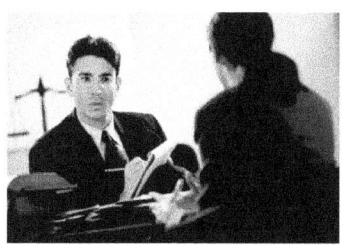

Chapter 7 Defenses

A patient has been injured; a suit is threatened or filed. The medical record, incident report, and statements by those involved in the incident are gathered by the defense attorney. The attorney then determines the most appropriate defense.

Statute of Limitations
- As described earlier, each state defines a time period for filing a suit. Depending on the state, the time period is based on when the plaintiff knew or should have known that an injury may have been caused by negligence.
- The statute is typically extended for a minor.
- An individual who approaches an attorney after the statute of limitations has expired will encounter difficulty securing agreement to file a suit.

Sovereign Immunity
- Certain county, municipal, city and state agencies may be protected from being sued for malpractice.
- Many states have abolished or restricted this common law doctrine.

Good Samaritan Law
- All states have enacted Good Samaritan Laws to encourage healthcare providers to stop and render help at the scene of an accident.
- In most states, the healthcare provider is protected from liability if care rendered is negligence, but the laws do not protect against gross misconduct or willful or wanton conduct that harms a person. [68]

- If a nurse receives a fee for services, the Good Samaritan statute cannot be used.

Case Example
After two days of difficulty breathing the patient, who was in his thirties, went to the emergency room of Provena St. Mary's Hospital. He was diagnosed with epiglottitis and admitted to the ICU. The plaintiff was later transferred to a regular medical floor where he experienced increased difficulty breathing. The man then stopped breathing and went into respiratory distress, leading to brain damage. A code blue was called when the respiratory distress occurred. An emergency room physician responded, but the plaintiff claimed that the man was without sufficient oxygen for forty-five minutes due to multiple unsuccessful attempts to insert a breathing tube. The plaintiff claimed that the nursing staff should have contacted the ear, nose, and throat physician treating the man while he was still in the ICU. The plaintiff also claimed that when a nurse contacted a hospital attending physician she failed to fully communicate the problems the man was experiencing.

The man was found to be disabled and a guardian of his estate was appointed. The hospital settled the case for $4.9 million. The ENT physician and his group settled for $1.75 million. The court dismissed claims against the emergency room physician who responded to the code blue, citing the Good Samaritan Act. That dismissal was appealed and the appeal was pending. [69]

Nursing Judgment
- Based on the information available at the time, the nurse made a judgment about how to handle a situation.
- The nurse was not gifted with hindsight (did not know there was going to be a negative outcome).

- This defense is effective only if the nurse followed the standard of care.
- The defense is often used in conjunction with the two schools of thought defense - there were two (or more) acceptable ways to perform a procedure. The nurse used reasonable judgment in selecting the approach and should not be held liable for the untoward outcome.

Comparative or Contributory Negligence
- The acts of the patient are examined to see if he or she caused or contributed to the injury.
- In some states, if the jury finds the patient was more than 50% at fault for the injury, no money will be awarded.
- If the jury finds the patient had some comparative negligence, the award is reduced by the percentage of liability of the patient.
- This defense is effective in some situations, such as a mentally competent patient not following the instructions of the ambulatory care nurse, such as coming in for care or going to an emergency department.
- Medical record documentation that described noncompliance by the patient that contributed to an injury is crucial for helping a defense attorney assert this defense.

Case Example
The plaintiff, age thirty-four, developed appendicitis while incarcerated in jail following arrest for assaulting his employer. The appendix ruptured. The plaintiff suffered pleurisy as a complication. The plaintiff claimed that the diagnosis and treatment of his appendicitis was delayed due to the actions of the nurse employee. The defendant claimed

that the nurse acted reasonably and that the plaintiff's symptoms were not consistent with appendicitis partly due to the plaintiff having a retrocecal appendix. The defendant also argued that the plaintiff contributed to any delay because he lied to the nurse about his condition. The plaintiff admitted this. A defense verdict was returned.

Disputed Facts
- A defense that is based on disputing facts focuses on proving the patient's version of events was wrong. For example, this may be used by referring to a recorded telephone conversation.
- The medical record's descriptions of care and events are heavily used in this type of defense.
- Independent witnesses may dispute the plaintiff's version of events.
- The plaintiff may be an unreliable witness. For example, an elderly person with dementia who fell may not be able to give an accurate description of what occurred.

Disputed Proximate Cause
- Sometimes the defense attorney may argue that there was no liability by the nurse, and even if the nurse was negligent, the actions of the nurse did not harm the patient.
- Negative outcomes can occur even in the absence of negligence.
- This defense is often used when a person is ill with a number of medical conditions, any of which may have caused the outcome as opposed to the actions of a nurse.
- Physician expert witnesses are often used to dispute proximate cause.

Assumption of the Risk
- The plaintiff, by agreeing to have a procedure or treatment performed, assumed the expressed, voluntary, or implied risks.
- This theory is based upon the informed consent of the patient. [70]

Patient Care was the Responsibility of Others
- The nurse may assert that he or she was not assigned to the patient at the time of the care.
- The nurse may assert that the physician (or another person) made the decisions in the care. [71]

Recognized Complication
- The injury could have occurred in the absence of negligence since it was a recognized complication of a procedure, according to expert witnesses and the medical literature.
- This defense is often used in surgical cases to explain the development of infection, lacerations of blood vessels and nerves, and punctures in the bowel.

Feedback Question
Review the case below and identify the type of defense the hospital attorney used.

Case Example
The plaintiff was admitted to the hospital with gastroesophageal reflux disease and a hernia. She had abdominal surgery later that day. After surgery she went to a regular room. In the early evening the nursing staff was called to a patient's room next door to the room occupied by the plaintiff. The staff found the plaintiff in the room with blood on her face and gown. Bruises appeared around her

eye. The staff escorted the plaintiff back to her own bed. In her room, they found a pool of blood on the side of the bed opposite the door.

Over the next several days, the hospital investigated to find out why the plaintiff, who was confused after the incident, had been wandering out of her room with blood on her face. Three possibilities were developed: a fall, a seizure or a beating. The plaintiff did not have a history of seizures and tests did not show any signs she had suffered one. The extent of her injuries seemed inconsistent with a fall. The treating physician through that the injuries were consistent with a beating, but doubted the plaintiff could have been beaten so severely without crying out. No one heard a struggle.

The plaintiff remembered nothing. The plaintiff claimed she had been a victim of a criminal assault and that the hospital was at fault for failing to protect her. The defendant claimed the nursing staff could not have any responsibility for a fall or a seizure and maintained that the plaintiff could not have been beaten without a noise which would have alerted the staff. A defense verdict was returned. [72]

Answer
This is a classic case of disputing the plaintiff's theory of how she was injured. The defense effectively disputed the theory that the staff was negligent for her injuries.

Let us try another one. What type of defense was used?

Case Example
The plaintiff's decedent, age seventy-two, was admitted to the hospital because of angina. During the admission, the cap of his IV became dislodged. The attending nurse swabbed the IV and replaced the cap, but did not attempt to replace

the IV itself. The decedent was discharged from the hospital but returned within eight hours with a methicillin-resistant staphylococcus aureas infection. He died of overwhelming sepsis, secondary to endocarditis caused by the infection. The plaintiff claimed the infection developed due to the dislodged IV cap. Simply swabbing the IV and replacing the cap did not eliminate contamination. The defendants claimed that the decedent had multiple IVs over the course of his admission. The MRSA bacteria could have entered through any of those IVs. The defendants argued that the plaintiff had no proof the IV in question was the source of the infection. The jury returned a $600,000 verdict. An appeal was expected. [73]

Answer
The defense disputed the proximate cause between the actions of the nurse and the infection.

Chapter 8 Legal Doctrines Pertinent to Nurse Administrators

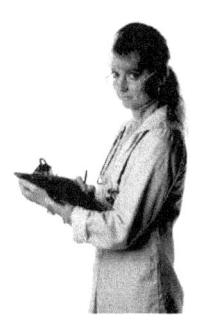

Hiring

- The nurse manager is responsible for hiring competent personnel.
- Employees are generally hired as "at-will" employees, meaning there is no written contract specifying a term of employment.
- The employer or the employee may terminate an at-will employee agreement without cause or notice.
- The at-will doctrine does not permit retaliation against an employee who acts as a whistleblower - who is testifying about his or her employer's acts, or is a union organizer. Nor does it permit termination based on discrimination because of race, sex, religion, sexual orientation or age.
- Nurse managers should consult with the Human Resources Department as to the facility's policies on hiring and checking references.
- Nurse managers should be aware of the questions that may not be asked in an interview which would violate state or federal anti-discrimination and employment laws. For example, do not ask women in child bearing years if they plan to have children, or ask about sexual orientation or religion of an individual.
- Federal regulations prohibit facilities from hiring individuals who have been found guilty of abuse, neglect, or mistreatment of a patient.
- Nursing home federal regulations require the facility to check the state nurse aide registry before hiring to identify an aide who has been reported for abuse.

- Federal law requires facilities to report to state licensing authorities any knowledge of legal proceedings against an employee that indicates unfitness to serve as a nurse aide or other facility staff. [74]
- The original copy of a nursing license should be reviewed. Some facilities copy the nurse's license for the permanent file; but some others are moving toward not keeping photocopies in order to reduce the risk of unauthorized use.
- A nurse manager may be found liable for negligent hiring when the facility knew or should have known the individual had a criminal background.

Case Example
A nurse hired as a registered nurse was working in a clinic shortly after becoming employed. She asked another staff member what an insulin syringe looked like. Becoming suspicious, the staff member contacted the nursing supervisor and nurse recruiter. When the new employee's file was pulled, it was determined that she had submitted a photocopy of her nursing license. She had pieced together two parts of a nursing license, and was in actuality a licensed practical nurse and not a registered nurse. The nurse recruiter learned the importance of requesting to see the original license. The nurse was terminated.

Case Example
The plaintiff's decedent, age twenty-three, had been born physically and mentally handicapped. In October 2000, an employee of defendant MedLink of Ohio, a home healthcare company, took the decedent to the defendant University Hospitals of Cleveland for dialysis treatment. The employee then left while the decedent had the treatment. During the

treatment the decedent pulled the catheter from her chest. A nurse found the decedent unresponsive and resuscitated her, but the decedent had suffered brain damage and she died a month and one-half later after her mother ordered the removal of the feeding tubes.

The plaintiff claimed that the MedLink employee had been instructed to sit with the decedent during the dialysis treatment because the decedent was known to have removed the chest catheter on prior occasions. The plaintiff also argued that the employee had a criminal record for felonious assault and MedLink was negligent in hiring the employee. The plaintiff claimed that University Hospital's employees failed to provide timely and appropriate treatment. The plaintiff claimed that the decedent's brain damage was due to air bubbles that triggered cardiac arrest due to the open catheter site. MedLink acknowledged that it had improperly hired the employee, but claimed that there was no guarantee that the outcome would have been any different if the employee had stayed with the decedent during the treatment.

MedLink also argued that the cardiac arrest could not have been prevented and there was no certainty as to what caused the cardiac arrest. University Hospitals contended that the staff did everything possible to save the decedent. According to Ohio Trial Reporter, a $6.1 million verdict was returned which included $3.1 million in compensatory damages with ninety percent liability assigned to MedLink and ten percent liability assigned to University Hospitals. The jury also awarded $3 million in punitive damages against MedLink only. The hospital reached a confidential settlement following trial and a motion for new trial by MedLink's insurer, AIG, was pending. [75]

Supervision

- Nurse managers may be involved in making patient care assignments, or may delegate this responsibility to charge nurses.
- The process of creating assignments involves knowing the skill levels and competencies of the staff and the needs of the patients.
- Nurse managers must know the state practice act and understand the tasks that can be safely delegated.

Consider the six rights of delegation:

- The right person with the appropriate skills should be asked to perform the care. The nurse manager must know the qualifications and competencies of the staff.
- The right task should be delegated for a specific patient. Complex tasks involving judgment should not be delegated to unlicensed personnel.
- Delegation should take place in the right circumstances, considering the available resources.
- Provide the right direction to the person, clearly defining the task, the limits and expectations.
- Provide the right supervision, which calls for knowing the qualifications of the staff, knowing the results of the delegated tasks, and evaluating performance. [76]
- Provide the right follow up to make sure the delegated task was done properly. [77]

The nurse manager or nurse acting in the delegating role may be liable if:

- Care is delegated to a nurse or unlicensed professional who is not qualified to perform the care.
- The unlicensed healthcare worker is asked to perform a nursing function: assessment, analysis, evaluation, the exercise of nursing judgment, and patient teaching.
- The unlicensed worker does not understand which concerning symptoms or data to report to a licensed nurse.
- The manager knew, or should have known, that supervision was needed and not provided.
- The manager does not take action to prevent injury when he or she was present and able to intervene.

Staffing
- A nurse manager is responsible for working with nursing administration to secure adequate staffing for the patient care setting.
- Nurse managers should be aware of any state or federal regulations that affect staffing or patient ratios, as well as mandatory overtime.
- When nurses from a unit are routinely pulled to another unit, sufficient cross training must be provided to assure a level of competency on the second unit.
- A nurse who is pulled to a different nursing area will be judged by how a reasonably prudent nurse working in that area would perform.
- Staffing decisions are based on the acuity of the patient, the qualifications of the available staff, and the availability of unlicensed personnel.
- A nurse manager may be liable for permitting patients to be admitted to a unit that is insufficiently staffed, or for failing to work with the facility

administration staff to assure sufficient nursing staff members are assigned to a unit.

Policies and Procedures

- It is common for nurse managers to participate in the drafting and review of policies and procedures.
- Policies and procedures should be based on evidenced-based practice, reviewed, and updated periodically.
- Ensure that staff can access policies and procedures at any time, whether in paper or electronic form.
- Maintain policies and procedures for a period of time as directed by administration so that they can be produced in the event of a lawsuit.
- Avoid including language in policies/procedures that sets unrealistic expectations. Do not promise that the patient will receive the highest level of care, when it may not be possible to always deliver it.
- Plaintiff attorneys may name nurse managers who had an active role in endorsing policies or procedures that were negligently drafted. For example, inclusion of interventions which research has shown to be ineffective or harmful, may constitute negligence.
- The nurse manager may be liable for failing to follow facility policy.
- If the facility sets a higher standard of care than is required by federal, state or other regulatory guidelines, the facility will be held to that higher standard.

Case Example

A nursing home set a policy that the family should be notified whenever a patient was involved in an incident, whether or not injury occurred. When the facility failed to notify the family of three falls, including one that resulted when the resident escaped from the facility, the plaintiff nursing expert testified that the facility failed to follow its own policy.

Case Example

The plaintiff's decedent, an eighty-seven year-old woman, sustained a skin tear on her leg in either late April or early May of 2003. The event was not noted in nursing records, however, until June 10, when the condition advanced to infection and a physician was notified. Antibiotics were administered on June 11. The decedent was sent to a wound care center for treatment on December 29. The leg was amputated on January 5, 2004. Gangrene set in and a second amputation was done. Unfortunately, the decedent contracted pneumonia and died on March 25, 2004. The plaintiffs claimed that the defendant's personnel caused the original injury by dropping a wheelchair footrest on the leg. The plaintiffs also asserted that employees failed to notify a physician in violation of state elder abuse laws. A state health department survey concluded that the defendant did not have a policy and procedure with regard to peripheral pulses. It failed to implement a policy on incident reporting for residents, it failed to implement a policy on skin tears and it repeatedly failed to provide weekly updates in the non-pressure skin condition report. The defense denied negligence, arguing that there was no clear evidence that an employee dropped a foot rest on the decedent's leg. It also asserted that a physician was promptly notified. Finally, the defense claimed that death was due to natural causes, including underlying circulatory problems and peripheral vascular disease. According to published accounts, the case settled in mediation for $400,000.[78]

Performance Evaluations

- Nurse managers should meet facility expectations regarding the timing of performance evaluations.
- Reviews should be based on objective information.
- Failure to undertake timely and objective performance evaluations may lead to a charge of discrimination when making promotion decisions.
- Evaluations should be reviewed by the employee, signed, and filed.

Impairment

- Healthcare providers are at risk for suffering from various forms of impairment from drugs, alcohol, fatigue, or aging-related cognitive decline.
- Cognitive and performance skills clouded by the effects of narcotics may contribute to patient injury. Substance abuse problems are prevalent in nursing, with the exact numbers difficult to establish.
- Substance abuse is one of the most frequent reasons that nurses are disciplined by the Board of Nursing.
- Recognition is growing that it is dangerous to stay awake for 24 hours or more; the impairment that results is similar to being inebriated.
- Medical errors are associated with fatigue. Fatigue contributes to impaired critical thinking. Twelve-hour shifts, which can extend even longer, contribute to errors and near errors.
- The night shift and rotating shifts are of particular concern in terms of performance. Fatigue, irritability, reduced performance, and decreased mental agility

may be present in some nurses working these hours. [79]

- The Institute of Medicine (IOM) concluded, "There is no evidence to suggest that any amount of training, motivation, or professionalism is able to overcome the performance deficits associated with fatigue, sleep loss, and sleepiness associated with circadian variations in alertness." The IOM concluded that the evidence related to prolonged work hours and fatigue was strong and recommended that state regulatory bodies prohibit nurses from working more than twelve hours in a twenty-four hour period and more than sixty hours per seven day period. [80]
- Impaired healthcare providers must be identified and treated (if the impairment is causing more than a transient problem).
- It is a nurse's responsibility to identify colleagues with substance abuse problems, yet this is difficult for many. It is especially difficult for nurses to report a peer, given the nature of nurses who often empathize with the problems of their colleagues.
- The nurse manager is charged with the responsibility to report impaired professionals.
- The impaired healthcare provider may face suspension and disciplinary action from a state licensing authority.
- Disciplinary action will trigger a report from the state licensing authority to the National Practitioner Data Bank. [81]
- Nurses often practice for several years with undiagnosed or unrecognized chemical dependency problems. It may take as long as five years before the nurse's addiction problem is discovered by others. Patients may have been endangered for this extended period of time. [82]

Discipline and Termination

- Facilities usually define a progressive disciplinary process, such as verbal warning, written warning, suspension, and termination.
- An employee may be disciplined for habitual tardiness, failure to call in when not coming to work, and other actions.
- Discipline following a medication or other error discourages reporting of such incidents. A non-punitive work environment encourages reporting of errors and near misses so that systemic errors may be identified and fixed.
- Blatant ignoring of policies and procedures, resulting in errors, may need to be addressed through discipline.
- Facility policies should define offenses which may result in termination. These generally include:
  - Lying.
  - Stealing.
  - Cheating.
  - Illicit drug use on the premises.
  - Hitting an employee or patient. [83]
  - Sexually assaulting an employee or patient.
- Precise and detailed documentation should be developed to justify a decision to terminate an employee. The file should record the progressive disciplinary actions taken to correct the situation, and the responses of the employee.
- Wrongful termination suits may be defended with this documentation. The facility's legal counsel should be consulted when appropriate.

The nurse manager:

- Should speak with Human Resources when a staff member's care is in question. This will provide guidance on how to implement the progressive disciplinary steps used in the facility.
- Has a responsibility to evaluate the care delivered by the nursing staff. If the nurse manager has concerns regarding patient safety, then the staff member is removed from providing direct patient care until the concerns are addressed.
- Should identify the needs of the nursing staff, such as more education, preceptorship, leadership, and development of advocacy skills.
- Must document concerns with patient care within the staff member's personnel file and a follow up plan of care with a timeline.

Fraud and Abuse

- The nurse manager may become aware of fraudulent practices being endorsed or undertaken by other healthcare providers.
- The fraud may involve altering records, concealing evidence, or submitting false claims for financial reimbursement, among other actions.
- Fraud is an intentional deception or misrepresentation that someone makes, knowing it is false, that could result in the payment of some unauthorized benefit. Abuse involves actions that are inconsistent with sound medical, business or fiscal practices.
- The primary difference between fraud and abuse is a person's intent. That is, did the person know he or she was committing a crime? [84]

In this billing fraud case, a physical therapist documented treatment given to a patient after his death. See the death certificate that follows.

®		SS NOTES
☒ Physical Therapy	☐ Occupational Therapy	☐ Speech Language Pathology

Patient's Name		Room # 607-1	Medical Record # 20104

DATE	NOTES MUST BE SIGNED WITH NAME AND CREDENTIALS
10/6/00	Resident not seen 2° illness.
10/13/00	Resident seen for short session 2° illness. Less alert than usual.
10/18/00	Resident seen for short session 2° his illness. He is less alert but able to communicate orientation X3 slowly but accurately.
10/29/00	Resident seen for short session 2° treatment by nursing.

STATE OF WISCONSIN
DEPARTMENT OF HEALTH AND FAMILY SERVICES
ORIGINAL CERTIFICATE OF DEATH
STATE FILING DATE
STATE DEATH NO.

Last	2 SEX M☒ F	3. SOC SEC NUMBER OF DECEDENT	4a PRONOUNCED DEAD DATE Mo Day Yr October 11, 2000	4b HOUR Hour 1:45 P M☒	5 BODY FOUND 24+ hours after death Y☐ N☒
7. DATE OF BIRTH Mo. Day Yr. February 15, 1928	8a. COUNTY OF DEATH Waukesha		8b DEATH OCCURRED INSIDE CITY, VILL. TOWNSHIP Waukesha		8c. (CHECK ONE) City☐ Vill. Twnshp ☒

Whistleblowing
Nurses who report wrongdoing through the proper administrative channels may pay a heavy price. They may be:
- harassed,
- demoted,
- given a poor evaluation,
- forced to leave, or
- professionally isolated.

Nurse managers who are considering becoming whistleblowers by reporting wrongdoing should consider these recommendations:

- Seek legal advice before taking action.
- Educate yourself on federal and state whistleblower protection laws, which prevent employers from taking retaliatory actions against nurses for reporting wrongdoing.
- Contact your state nurses association for answers and clarifications.
- Create a paper trail by documenting episodes of abuse or fraud, including dates, times, and outcomes. Make copies of all documentation and keep them in a secure location.
- When reporting wrongdoing, stick to the facts and follow your organization's chain of command.
- Reach out for help from your professional nursing organizations, state attorney general, Department of Defense Inspector General, Congress, and other organizations.
- Send all documentation to outside agencies by certified mail so you can verify receipt of materials.
- Be professional when dealing with your organization's administration and outside agencies. [85]

Captain of the Ship

- The doctrine of captain of the ship is used to place full responsibility for the care of the patient on the surgeon in the operating room.
- This doctrine makes the surgeon responsible for all actions of all those present in the room during the operation, including nurses, technicians, and physicians.

- Most states have abandoned this doctrine and hold individuals responsible for their own actions.

 Scan this QR code for video highlights of a presentation by Pat Iyer on documentation.

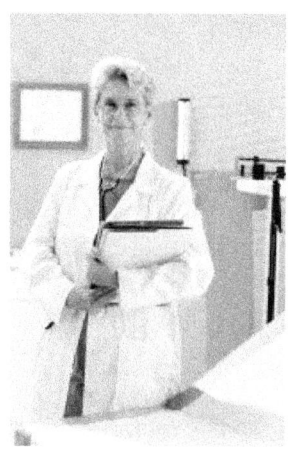

Chapter 9 Nursing Documentation

Do you ever feel like you have lots of roles? As a nurse, you are receptionist, patient and family educator, patient advocate, housekeeper, dietician, and communicator with physicians. You are at the center of the healthcare wheel. Some of the choices you take on voluntarily; others are thrust upon you. You may wonder how you can serve so many masters. Life as a nurse becomes a juggling act, and maintaining your balance is the key to survival. The medical record is one of your masters.

Like you, the medical record has a lot of roles. It is designed for communication, regulatory compliance and as a legal document. It provides continuity of care from home to medical office, shift to shift, unit to unit and from one facility to another. The record is used to justify the level of care, and to terminate coverage when the patient has reached a level of progress. It is used to verify something was done and to reconstruct events.

Documentation is an essential part of nursing practice. It changes periodically with trends in health care, patient safety efforts and regulatory standards. There are invisible people looking over your shoulder when you chart.

Entities that Govern Charting
The American Academy of Ambulatory Nursing has a standard that addresses the need to document and share plans with team members, including the patient and caregivers. The ambulatory care nurse uses documentation

tools that support continuity of care within a multidisciplinary environment. [86] When we look at liability issues, it's the standards that drive how people evaluate your charting.

Case Example
I received a call a couple of years ago from a nursing educator at a hospital who said that The Joint Commission surveyor walked in to do a survey and she decided to follow the flow of the patient through the facility.

This particular patient was in the endoscopy area and was having a GI procedure. The Joint Commission surveyor looked at the chart. The chart said that the procedure went according to the plan and that there were no complications and normal findings. The problem was that the patient was still in the preop holding area when the chart was written by the physician with that note. The procedure had not even been done yet.

You can imagine the reaction. The hospital was very close to being cited and sanctioned because of that note by that physician, so they brought me in to talk about documentation. I don't know what happened to the physician who wrote that note, but I would imagine that there were some repercussions.

Department of Health
The Department of Health also has a series of standards that govern charting. You may have seen the standards and the impact on the clinical units when the standards are being changed.

Factors that Affect Nursing Documentation

There are lot of factors that affect nursing documentation and trends that will direct how you chart. One of the issues is increased consumer awareness. Your parent may call you and say, "You know, I was just checking on the Internet. I think that I need to have surgery and I'm thinking that maybe I'll go to this hospital because they are well known for that particular procedure," or "I was just checking on the Internet and you know I might be having these side effects of this medication and I'm thinking maybe it's due to the medication. I should be taking a different medication." Or you'll hear people talking in the grocery store about healthcare issues. You'll see in a women's magazine, Women's Today or Ladies' Home Journal, "10 things that you can do to lose weight" or "10 risks of cardiovascular disease". It is so pervasive that it is hard to think of a person who is not educated on some of those basic principles.

There's more awareness now on the part of consumers about the risks in health care and the patient safety issues that they should be paying attention to.

There are more forms, details, and questions being asked. It is difficult to fill out a lot of paperwork given the demands of patient care. The amount of time that's available for charting has been compressed. Just the amount of work is increased for all the nurses because we're actually doing so many different jobs in addition to our own job. There is a lot of stress added to the role of a nurse.

The reality is that we can do all those other things but it's not the best use of our time. We should be assessing and evaluating. The biomedical people can't do that. They can change the battery on the equipment but they can't complete a care plan or figure out that subtle change in a patient that requires a call to the doctor because something is happening to that patient. Likely you've been in that situation where you've seen an emergency developing and you know that you've got to put the pieces together to get somebody in to look at the patient.

Never Events
Never events are outcomes that should never occur in health care. The Centers for Medicare and Medicaid Services will not reimburse hospitals for care that leads to the development of a never event. Never events include things like a foreign object left in the body. Nothing thrills a plaintiff attorney more than an x-ray that shows a clamp in the abdomen. Nothing scares the OR nurses more than hearing about those things, doing an operation on the wrong limb, or on the wrong patient.

Case Example
A friend of mine, who works at a very large hospital in Boston, told me that a couple of the OR nurses were taking a woman down to the operating room for a neck operation. She was taking care of this patient and said, "Wait a minute, that patient is not having surgery." The techs replied, "Oh yes, we've got to take her to the OR; she is going to the OR." They picked up the wrong patient out of the bed and were planning to take her down to the operating room for a laminectomy on the neck.

Another never event is performing surgery on the wrong side, and that's why we do time outs in the OR. We double check whenever there's an invasive procedure that we've got the right person. The development of a stage 3 or a stage 4 pressure ulcer in the hospital is also a never event.
Several private payers echoed the stance of CMS and refused to pay for never events. These insurance companies said, "If it's good enough for the government to not have to pay, it's good enough for us not to have to pay either."

There are urinary tract infections and IV catheter-related infections that fit on that never event list. A person who gets burned particularly in the operating room as a potential source for burns or receives an electric shock, is electrocuted; that's also a never event. The issue of falls is tricky as a never event because there are some people who fall without there being any negligence on the part of the providers. There is a lot of debate going on in the reimbursement world about whether every fall should be denied in terms of payment. There's no final word on this issue.

From a liability perspective, we know that people will be told, "Don't get out of bed without calling for help; your call bell is right over here; be sure to ask for assistance," and there are people who will disregard all of that. Your best bet when you provide that kind of instruction to a patient and the patient falls is to be sure to document that you warned the patient to not get out of bed without help. That will prevent lawsuits from being filed.

Whether that's reimbursable or non-reimbursable care may be influenced by whether the patient was alert and oriented and was instructed or was the patient confused. You provided the instruction, but the patient wasn't capable of remembering or following that instruction. So then what else did you do?

Providing the patient with incompatible blood is another never event. There have been horrible cases of people getting the wrong blood when somebody checked the ID band or checked the numbers at the nurse's station instead of looking at the patient's ID band. It's crucial that you know who you are infusing blood into. The band numbers have to match the blood bag, which have to match the chart. All those numbers match up.

The list of never events gets added to. From the patient's safety perspective, the good news is that when we focus on these things, we make inroads. We have nurses who are better at washing their hands. We have doctors who are better about ordering that Foleys be removed quickly after surgery. We are better in identifying people in the hospital OR before performing surgery.

You still see headlines of a patient who was brought into the hospital when a wrong kidney was removed. You still see that today, but you see fewer of them, so we are making a difference with these issues. And everyone is focusing on patient's safety.

The Institute for Healthcare Improvement identifies patient safety issues, as does the National Quality Foundation, CMS, and Joint Commission. There are lots of people asking, "Where can we improve quality? What can we do to improve the issues that cause these kinds of errors?" Nursing is a huge part of this whole campaign.

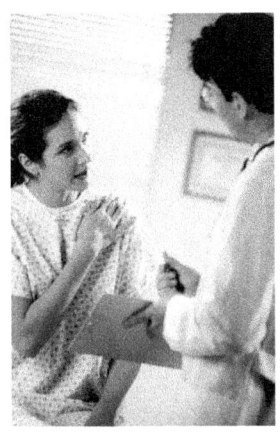

Chapter 10 Creating Bullet Proof Nursing Documentation

Attorneys and expert witnesses review documentation to evaluate how the standard of care was fulfilled. They may ask:

- Did you collect the appropriate assessment data?
- Did you identify the problem?
- Did you come up with a plan?
- Did you carry out the plan?
- Did you update the plan when the person's condition changed?

Remember that the key is to look at the nursing process and the patient. We don't have all the same needs. Look at the risk issues in your particular clinical area and make sure that you're addressing them.

The plan of care should identify the priority, individualized, current and updated issues for the patient. As an example, if somebody is at risk for falls, are the risk factors identified?

Timing and Dating Records

When we look at charting and timing of charting, a couple of issues come up. One of them is multi page flow sheets. They are used in ambulatory care centers, medical surgical and critical care units. It can sometimes be very difficult to piece them together if a date is not written on each page. Without a date on every sheet, the reviewer is challenged when trying to match signatures and handwriting to figure out how the flow sheet goes together.

Dating flow sheets is important. Dating pages when you're manually writing notes is important or writing the word "continued" at the top of the page.

Late Entries

Late entries are scrutinized by plaintiff attorneys. These entries are typically written after a bad outcome has occurred. They usually are a "cover-my-behind" note. Late notes have important details that you should've charted at that time. The correct way of adding them is to put in today's date and say "late entry for" and then the date that you should've charted the information. The sooner you can chart it, the better. Remember the purpose of the charting is to communicate important information from one shift to the next, so the sooner you add the note, the better. When is it too late to put in a late entry - at the time that the plaintiff attorney already has the chart, for example? That would be too late. As soon as possible, as soon as you realized that something was not charted, it should be added.

I've seen several charts of people who got transferred to the critical care unit and the medical surgical nurses didn't have a chance to do their charting before the patient was gone. In one case, the nurse who was asked to complete her chart after the patient was transferred, put in information that was inaccurate. That was detected in the analysis of the case. There's always that question of what happened. What were those events that led up to the transfer? So the sooner that information is in the chart, the better.

Format of Charting – Label Chart with Patient's Name

Additionally, the format of charting is important. Label pages with the patient's name. In an emergency, you may grab a paper towel or write on the sheet that is on the stretcher or the bed. That information all needs to be brought into the medical record.

Errors can occur when staff members label pages. Probably 1 out of every 50 charts that I review as a legal nurse consultant has a page in it that is stamped with a different patient's name. Sometimes, that's a stamping error or identification error and sometimes it's a sheet that should have been in the other patient's chart but ended up in our patient's chart. This is a risk when you care for people with the same first or last names. The difficulty is that there might be information documented on that sheet that is missing from the other person's chart but also influences your patient's chart.

Case Example
I vividly remember the medical record of a 79-year-old woman who had a fractured hip. A note was written by a student nurse and cosigned by her instructor that said they sat down and counseled the patient about methadone treatment, and I thought, "A 79-year-old patient with a fractured hip on methadone treatment? I don't think so." The note referred to the sex of the patient as a male. Always be sure when you're picking up a chart that you do indeed have the right chart. Look at it before you pick it up. Look at it after you close it. If you do make an error and chart on the wrong chart, you can draw a line through and say "mistaken entry" and you're not going to be faulted for that. I see that frequently people will cross off a line or an entry and just indicate it as a charting entry. But it does create a concern among the attorneys of how careful we are with charting if we're charting on the incorrect patient.

Cosigning Notes
Cosigning notes is typically done by instructors with students. If you are ever asked to cosign a note, it means that you are accepting responsibility for the accuracy of that note.

Identifying Personnel

If you report something to a nursing supervisor, put the name of the nursing supervisor in the note. I recommend that you use people's names in medical records. This helps to establish accountability. That helps to show that you fulfilled your responsibility and it also helps to identify that person if there's a question later on. Without an identifying the name, it is difficult to reconstruct who that person was.

Record Care You Provide

In another example, you may start an IV for another nurse. Who is then responsible for documenting the start of the IV? Is it the person who put it in or the nurse of the patient? You may do this either way as long as you identify the name of the person who actually inserted the IV. Document the gauge, the vein and the number of attempts.

Blanks on Forms

Blanks on a form raises the question of why there are blanks.

- What happened?
- Was the information overlooked?
- Was it omitted?
- Was it not applicable?

Indicate, if you can, why those areas are not filled in.

Illegible Handwriting

In some states, there is a regulation that says if your charting is illegible, you have to provide a transcription at the request of an attorney. You have to sit down and type it up. There are some physicians and nurses who are asked to do this in their deposition. Illegible handwriting is a huge source of error, aside from the legal issues.

I can't tell you the number of times that I've sat in a nurse's station and I've heard somebody holding a handwritten order sheet say, "What do you think it says?" "What's your opinion on this?" We shouldn't be playing guessing games when it comes to the names of medications and dosages and tests. I think that you will gradually see a reduction in that kind of a question because of the use of computerized documentation, but it can't come soon enough.

I know we may be in a hurry when we chart. We often don't take the time to sit down and review our records after we chart them, but if you did, you might pick up some spelling and grammatical errors. Some of the spelling that I have seen in reviewing charts is, frankly, creative, but it does make you wonder, is the chart fulfilling its obligation to communicate clearly?

Handwriting, zeros, and dosages are huge source of concern. What does the order say?

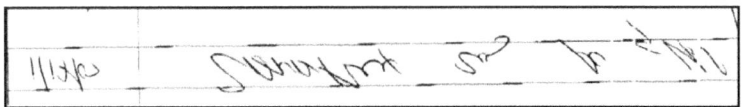

What's the drug and dosage? The dosage could be 2; it could be 20. The nurse who shared this order with me saw it as 20. It was actually 2. The nurse administered Zanaflex 20 mg. There was no harm done to the patient from the 20 mg, but the nurse ended up being referred to the board of nursing for making a transcription error. I worked with him to provide education on medication errors.

Here is another order. What does this order say?

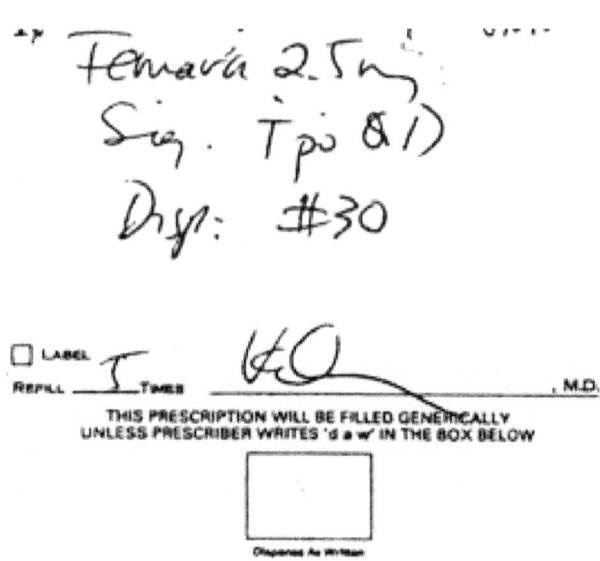

Femara 2.5mg
Sig. Tpo QD
Disp: #30

☐ LABEL
REFILL __I__ Times _____ , M.D.

THIS PRESCRIPTION WILL BE FILLED GENERICALLY
UNLESS PRESCRIBER WRITES 'd a w' IN THE BOX BELOW

Dispense As Written

The doctor intended to order Femara. The pharmacist read it as Premarin and gave it to a woman with uterine cancer who was not supposed to receive estrogen. The pharmacist repeated the dispensing error twice before the problem was detected.

Day 0	Prehydrate c̄ 125cc D5.5NS + 3.5g Mannitol + 8 mEq MgSO₄/L over 2 hours.	✓
	Zofran 1mg in 25ml D5W over 20 min q 4° × 2 doses then q 8° thereafter (first dose at least 20min ā Cisplatin)	✓
	Cisplatin 204mg + Mannitol 3.5g in NS to total 350cc over 6 hours	✓

The above figure shows an order for cisplatin. This was a case involving a 9-month-old infant who was supposed to receive 20.4 mg, but instead received 204 mg. When the order was transcribed, the decimal disappeared. When the order went down to the pharmacy to be filled, the pharmacists overlooked the black box warning on the package insert. The manufacturer recommended double-checking any dosage that fell into the range included in the 204 mg dose.

Two pharmacists checked the order but didn't pick this up and supplied it to the nursing unit. The child received the chemotherapy and died 2 days later. The toxicology studies found toxic levels of cisplatin in his blood. The pathologist also found on autopsy that the child had metastatic cancer in his adrenals. So from a damages perspective, this case of the death of a 9-month old infant wasn't really worth that much. However, there is a case law in New Jersey, where this overdose occurred, that says if a family member witnesses the malpractice, that person can file a claim for the damages that person suffered. The child's mother was in the room when the chemotherapy began, so she witnessed the error that killed her child. That transformed the value of a claim from $200,000 to over a million dollars.

Abbreviations
Abbreviations are imported with residents and interns or with doctors or nurses from other facilities. Healthcare providers make up their own abbreviations, which adds to miscommunication and medical errors.

The Joint Commission came up with a "do-not-use abbreviation list." The list has cut down rather significantly on the use of those unauthorized abbreviations. The Joint Commission highlighted abbreviations like U for unit or qd for every day. They also targeted the use of trailing zeros, such as 3.0. Also, instead of writing .5, the healthcare provider should write 0.5.

Bias

When we talk about bias, those are the words that you should not put in the chart about a particularly difficult patient. These words show your attitude towards the patient: "drunk", "obnoxious" or "irritating".

Using the word "demanding" to describe a patient is better than stating the patient is "irritating" which has a judgment call. Words that show bias make a reviewer wonder if the patient received good quality care. If your nursing entry comes under the scrutiny of a plaintiff attorney, he may say, "Clearly, you didn't like this patient because you used those words and therefore, the outcome that was obtained was because you didn't like the patient." Biased words imply that we are not providing objective care.

Translators

We have a huge issue in a multicultural area with communication. Many facilities use an outside translation service with a person on the other end of the phone. The interpreter relays messages between the nurse and the patient. The challenges relate to communicating across the language barrier and being able to share significant information.

If you obtain information through an interpreter, document this person's name.

Questioning Orders

The Joint Commission collects data on sentinel events and the factors that lead to errors. The number one issue is always communication. If you stop and think about how challenging it is to communicate, just within our nursing world, you can see the potential for errors. The potential for miscommunication increases when we mix in accents, language barriers, and fatigue.

Failure to question an inappropriate order probably causes more liability for nurses than any other aspect of what we've been talking about. Lots of cases that I've been involved in revolve around what the nurse told the doctor and how the doctor responded when there was an emerging problem. The whole realm of communication between doctors and nurses or nurses and other healthcare professionals is fraught with potential problems. The lawsuit may delve into what was ordered. What did the nurse say to the person who wrote the order? You are the final safeguard between an inappropriate or incorrect order and the patient. There's nobody after you.

As a nurse, you should step in and say, "Did you mean to write this order?" or "That dose seems too high," or "You wrote down 'elevate the right leg,' but it was the left leg that was operated on." When you step in and ask questions, you provide a very important safety net.

Chain of Command

The chain of command is a difficult issue. It's one that creates a lot of trouble when the nurse needs to act as a patient advocate and seek help for a patient.
You should be very knowledgeable about how to use the chain of command in your ambulatory care setting.

- What do you do when you've got a concern about a patient?
- How far do you take it?
- Who do you take it to?
- What do you chart about it?

Every facility typically has a chain of command policy that addresses this issue in terms of who to notify. The important thing to keep in mind as the overriding issue, is that we're all of us are patient advocates and have a responsibility to speak up when we see something that needs to be addressed. There are three reasons that nurses or other healthcare professionals typically give as to why the chain of command failed:

1. I didn't want to speak up because I was afraid it would affect my relationship with the physician.
2. I knew there was a problem and I told the physician but he didn't do anything about it.
3. I knew there was a problem and I told my nursing supervisor but I don't know what happened after that.

All of these reasons are unacceptable for not following the chain of command. Once you identify a problem, you need to continue to follow the problem until it is resolved. Your charting should reflect what you reported and did to act as a patient advocate.

Recording Changes in Condition

One of the liability issues that arise in ambulatory care lawsuits is documenting changes in condition. If these condition changes are concerning, what did you do about them? Nurses may be questioned during an investigation of an incident, or in a deposition. The questioning goes like this:

- "You picked up these symptoms; what did you do about them?
- Did you contact the physician?
- If the physician didn't respond the way that you expected, what did you do then?"

There has been a lot of talk about the principles of crew resource management, about bringing the safety of the airlines into health care. There are some pilots who are making a very good living teaching people about teamwork. The principle of teamwork is gaining acceptance in health care but there is still much to be done. We still have the hierarchical issue, "I'm the doctor; you are the nurse." Until nurses are fully respected as part of the healthcare team, and we earn that respect, we will see situations where intimidation causes nurses to clam up. That's the danger in health care - not speaking up.

It is the astute nurse who questions the physician who has overlooked something who saves a patient's life. You are charged with the responsibility to be a patient advocate. Remember, if you ever have the sense that something is going wrong, don't ever allow intimidation to prevent you from speaking up. It is better to be told, "He is okay, I'm aware of it," than to not ask the questions.

Delay in Treatment/Failure to Rescue
Another issue that comes up frequently in lawsuits is delays or gaps in treatment. For example, there may be a delay in performing surgery or doing a diagnostic test. Even if the CAT scan is ordered stat, the department may not be able to accommodate the patient. You may be told, "Even if it's a stat, we'll get to you when we get to you." You would document that you contacted them and that the patient is waiting for the CAT scan and that there's a backup and the department is aware of the stat order.

Your charting should reflect the attempts you made to facilitate the treatment, and the reasons for the delay. For example, if a patient calls the physician office requesting an appointment, your documentation should describe your attempts to secure an appointment for the next available time. Also, you should document your directive to the patient to go to an emergency department if the symptoms warrant immediate evaluation.

Delay in treatment is a liability issue that people are increasingly focusing on because of the fragility of our healthcare population. When we look at the issues of failure to rescue, we're talking about the inability to save a patient's life when concerning symptoms begin to develop and a complication is diagnosed. Nurses are typically the first people who detect complications and concerns, although they're not the only ones.

It's not enough to have plenty of staff and plenty of experienced staff if the experienced staff members don't mobilize the resources when they're necessary. There's increased risk of patient injury when there is a delay in recognizing and acting on symptoms.

Read Back of Telephone or Verbal Orders

So far I have stressed the importance of communication between healthcare professionals, the importance of documenting, and what you are reporting to other providers about a patient. You should be familiar with the read back of verbal orders and telephone orders, and document that you have done that. Read back of orders has prevented a lot of medication errors and other treatment errors. As a nurse, you are confirming with the prescriber, "Is this what you want the patient to receive?"

Allergies

Documentation of allergies is a huge issue. In my opinion, you can't chart them in enough places. Also the nurse must use critical thinking about this patient being is allergic to a medication. If a patient is allergic to one cephalosporin, for example, should the patient get another cephalosporin? Hopefully, that is picked up in the pharmacy, but sometimes it is an issue that is picked up in the nursing unit.

Case Example

I was involved in a case of a woman who was allergic to prednisone. She had a psychotic reaction to prednisone, which was given to her for asthma, after an orthopedic surgery. She had an external fixator on her wrist, and when she became psychotic, she was banging her wrist into the window in her room. She disrupted all of the hardware. The doctor discharged her and sent her home to let her heal. The orthopaedic surgeon admitted her to the hospital for the repair surgery. When she came in the second time, the internal medicine doctor ordered another form of prednisone. The allergy was written on the medication order sheet: she is allergic to prednisone, but the nurse did not think of Solu-Cortef as related to the prednisone and missed that. The patient received Solu-Cortef and she became psychotic again and was banging her wrist for the second time until the orthopedic surgeon said, ""That's it, I'm done." He refused to attempt to repair her arm a third time. The case settled out of court.

Noncompliance

If you give instructions to the patient and the patient doesn't follow them, you are likely not to be considered liable if there is a bad outcome. Juries believe that people should follow instructions. That's the belief that we have in our culture. If the nurse says, "Be sure to get your blood checked for clotting while you are on Coumadin", the patient's supposed to listen. I'm talking about the alert, oriented person who doesn't follow instructions. If the telehealth nurse asks the patient to come to the office or go to an urgent care center, and the patient refuses, this needs to be documented.

Charting in an Emergency
It's easy to put charting aside when you're dealing with a crisis and that's important. The focus is always on the patient first. It's a very valid defense to say I was focused on the patient's needs; I didn't do the charting at the same time; my first priority was the patient. That's a great response when questioned by a plaintiff attorney, but it's very important to put that information in the chart at a point where it's convenient and when it will be of value to the clinical staff taking care of the patient.

Mistaken Entries
Correct a mistaken entry by drawing a single line through it. Date, time and initial the change and provide an explanation of the change, such as "wrong patient".

Inappropriate Comments
Don't criticize other healthcare providers through the chart. This is also a fruitful ground for plaintiff attorneys. Defense attorneys cringe when they see comments in the medical record of staff members being critical of each other. The pointing of fingers just makes it easier for the plaintiff attorney to figure out where the liability resides.

Incident Reports
In some states, the plaintiff's attorney is allowed to see an incident report. These reports are scrutinized by attorneys, expert witnesses, risk managers, insurance claims adjusters and others involved in the litigation process.

Incident reports should be:

- Factual, detailing only what was seen and heard, and not contain speculation.
- Completed in a timely manner.
- Inclusive of an evaluation of the patient's condition performed by the licensed practitioner - physician, nurse practitioner, or physician's assistant.
- Devoid of recommendations for what should have been done differently.
- Promptly passed on to the next person in the chain of individuals required to review them.

Incident reports are not discoverable until a suit has been filed, but once the suit has been filed, in some states, they get turned over pretty frequently. Most incident report use a format with check offs. Avoid writing an essay, finger pointing or comments like, "This never would have happened if they had given us more staffing."

Just very objectively write the facts. The same facts belong in the medical record. The incident report information should be identical to the information that's in the medical record describing what happened. If an incident occurs and there's nothing in the chart, the plaintiff attorney might be able to allege that there was cover up; there was an attempt to conceal or hide what happened.

Documenting IVs and Blood Administration

When it comes to IVs and blood, I've already mentioned documenting the IV insertion details. When you're giving IMs, be sure to document the location of the IM. More medications are now being given by the IV route eliminating the IM route. This avoids the risks of nerve damage, but we still give IMs or subcutaneous injections occasionally and it's important to write the site.

If that patient develops a hematoma or nerve damage at the site, you want to make sure that it's not your injection that's going be considered the one that did the damage. You used the left leg site; the problem was in the right leg. You won't be brought in as a defendant if you can identify that you gave the injection in the site that was not affected.

Confidentiality of Medical Records

Do not bring home confidential information from your worksite. A friend of mine told me about a nurse on the nursing unit who had an unpleasant relationship with her landlord. She put out her garbage too early and the landlord went down to the curb and got the garbage out and went through it. He found patient care flow sheets or worksheets which he then took out of the garbage. He marched down to her employer's office in the hospital and said, "Look what this nurse is throwing out in the garbage."

Case Example

In another case that relates to confidentiality of information, the plaintiff became a patient of Internal Medicine Associates. He accumulated an unpaid debt to the group of $326. The defendant (Internal Medicine Associates) hired an attorney to collect on the debt. The defendant supplied the attorney with copies of billing statements which listed the plaintiff's name, address, phone number, social security number and date of birth. The information also listed the plaintiff's last diagnosis as being HIV positive. A year later, the attorney filed a small claims case against the plaintiff to collect on the unpaid bill. The attorney attached the billing statements as exhibits to the complaint. All of the plaintiff's identifying information, along with his HIV status, was in the exhibits. Internal Medicine Associates won the court case.

An attorney for the plaintiff sent the defendant's attorney a letter pointing out the disclosure of the plaintiff's HIV status. A motion was filed with the court to have the offending exhibit sealed, which was granted. The exhibit was part of the public record for six months. The plaintiff alleged that the Internal Medicine Associates' action in disclosing his HIV status was negligence.

The case went to trial. The defendant argued there were no damages and that the disclosure was not widely broadcast and had been sealed. The defendant also claimed it was the attorney's responsibility to redact (hide) the offending information. The jury returned at $1.25 million verdict. A post-trial settlement resulted in a recovery of $250,000. [88]

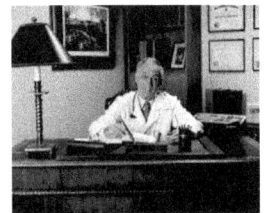

Chapter 11 Tampering with Medical Records

Tampering with records is not sloppy charting; it is not careless charting; it is not forgetting to put in some details about care. It is a deliberate attempt to change the medical records, to alter them to hide or conceal something. All of us at times, whether because of distraction or fatigue, will accidentally leave material out of a medical record. Tampering is done for a malicious intent. This is falsification of records. If you omit something or you forget something, and this is an honest mistake, that is not falsifying records.

There are people who have deliberately omitted information to hide something that has happened, but the true falsification or tampering, or spoliation of evidence is the legal term, is done deliberately for a malicious reason by the person who is changing the chart.

Adding to an Existing Record

Adding to an existing record at a later date is considered tampering with medical records. I saw a chart of a patient who came to a hospital from a nursing home. The physician squeezed in the entry here to say "bedsore on back." This inserted entry immediately popped out because it did not fit in on the line.

Placing Inaccurate Information into the Record

If healthcare providers put in inaccurate information into the record, it's considered tampering with records. Consider an incident report of a nursing home resident who fell out of bed. It stated that the patient fell from the bed, sustained swelling on the left side of the head, and a small skin tear on the left forearm. The bed was in the low position and there were mats on the floor. But the autopsy report showed subdural and subarachnoid hemorrhages. It showed a cerebral shift and it showed a fracture of the cervical spine, and the physician who was involved in looking at this said, "These injuries are not compatible with the gentle roll off of the bed onto mats. This was a more substantial fall than that."

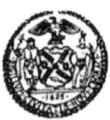

OFFICE OF CHIEF MEDICAL EXAMINER
CITY OF NEW YORK

REPORT OF AUTOPSY

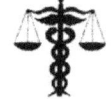

Name of Decedent: ███████████   M.E. Case #: ~~Q0004060~~

                                          ~~Q000+900~~

Autopsy Performed by: ███████████   Date of Autopsy: Dec. 1, 2000

CAUSE OF DEATH: BLUNT IMPACT INJURIES OF HEAD AND NECK
                         WITH SUBDURAL AND SUBARACHNOID
                         HEMORRHAGES, CEREBRAL SHIFT AND
                         FRACTURE OF CERVICAL SPINE. THIS IS A TRUE COP'
                                                    Office of the Chief Medical Examine
                                                    This record cannot be released withou
                                                    prior consent from the Office of Chie
MANNER OF DEATH: ACCIDENT. (FELL FROM BED). Medical Examiner. New York City, N.Y

I worked on a case involving a New York woman who was in the hospital for 7 months. The hospital's policy said that they should document the exact time the patient was turned. For 7 months, the patient was never turned at a time other than 1, 3, 7, 9 and 11. Sometimes the nurses left out the times all together, but there was no time other than those times charted for 7 months. She ended up with a stage IV pressure sore. Her daughter took her home and healed up the pressure sore in 3 months at home by turning her every 2 hours. This case settled at the court house as the trial was about to begin.

1-3-5-7	1-3-5-7	1-3-5-1	1-3-5-1	1-3-7	1-3-5-7
9-11-1-3	9-11-1-3	7-11-3	5-11-13	9-1-1-3	9-1-1-3
5,7,9,11				5-7-9-11	

I have occasionally encountered nurses who have thought that they could chart before they give the care and I've already given you the example of the physician who charted the endoscopy before the procedure was done. But I've met nurses, specifically in the recovery room areas, who took care of open-heart patients all the time, so they knew how the patient was going come out of the OR with all the lines. To save time, the nurses started writing out the notes, describing all the lines. They began charting before the patient even arrived in their area. That is considered tampering with records because its charting information before the care is actually rendered.

In another case, I saw a flow sheet that described antibiotics being started for a person who had wounds. The date on the flow sheet is 12/27; the order for the antibiotics is 12/30.

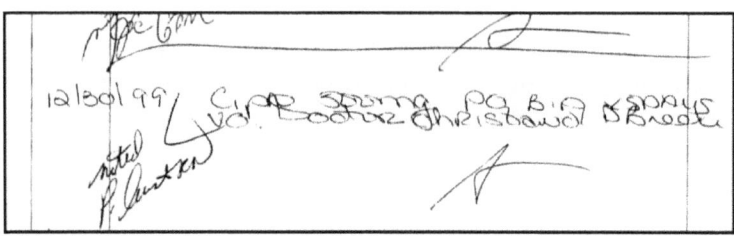

Omitting Significant Information

If you leave out significant information, that is tampering. Remember we're talking about something that is clinically significant and not a simple charting error.

Case Example

I worked on a case of a man who went in for a cervical laminectomy. He was on his third day postop and a nursing assistant came in to get him out of bed. She put a walker in front of him. She weighed about 100 pounds and he was 6-foot 4-inches and weighed 240 pounds. He said to her, "It took 3 people to get me up this morning," and she said, "Don't worry, I can do it." He got up; his knees buckled; he fell down. When he landed on the floor, the plug that was in his neck popped out and banged the spinal cord. The day shift nurse wrote nothing about the fall when he hit the floor with the nursing assistant.

There was nothing in this note that described an incident. It wasn't documented anywhere. Nobody was notified. There was no incident report. The only way that we knew that it happened was that there was a physical therapy student who wrote a note. She wrote that the patient "fell to the floor with nursing when transferring and he was complaining of a sharp pain like a jolt that forces him to buckle both legs, transferred back to bed with maximum assistance x3." See next page for the note.

The patient developed numbness and tingling later that night. He told the night nurse he could not move his toes and he was having trouble with sensation. She said to him, "That's okay, just use the extremities that you still have left." She wrote it in the nurse's notes.

By 7 o'clock in the morning, he was paralyzed from his nipple level down. The doctor, who didn't know that he was having changes in sensation, immediately took him to surgery, but it was too late, the cord was damaged. This was a case that was settled out of court.

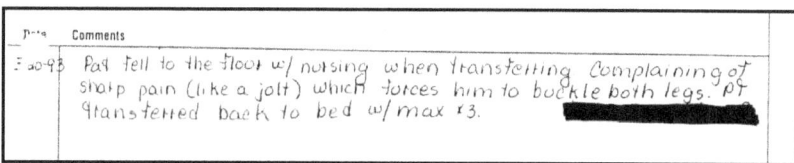

Occasionally, and I see it more in physician offices than I've seen it in hospitals, a physician will rewrite an entry or rewrite an office note after getting bad results, and then go back and look at the chart.

Altering Dates
In another lawsuit, the medical record contained a request for a swallowing evaluation that was ordered for a patient who was choking. The date was changed from February to March after the patient had a choking episode. The staff member did this to make it look as if the swallowing

evaluation did not sit there for a month with no action taken on it. See next page for the altered date.

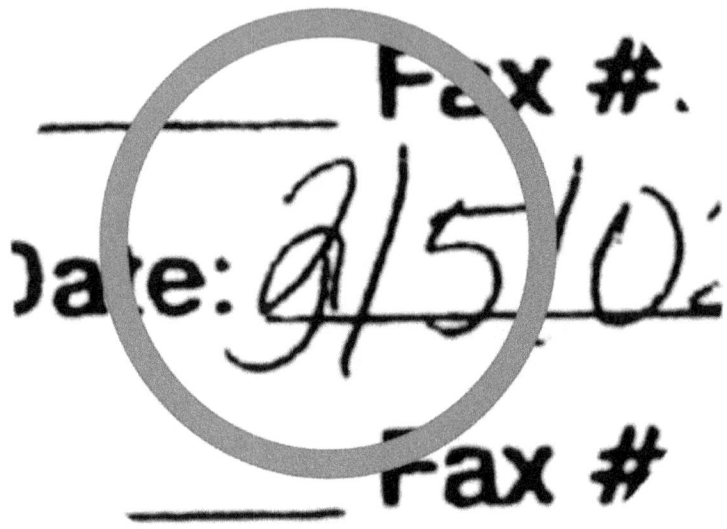

Destroying records

Destroying records by shredding, burning or discarding is tampering with records. I heard of a nursing home administrator who actually testified in his deposition that a dog came in his office and ate the medical records.
In another legal case, the nurses in the facility documented that they spilled liquid and accidentally destroyed the nurses' notes. They destroyed the care plans and the medication administration records, but they didn't destroy anything that wasn't important in terms of liability. The reality is that it's unusual for liquid to selectively destroy the parts of the chart that are most important in terms of defending or creating problems for the nurses.

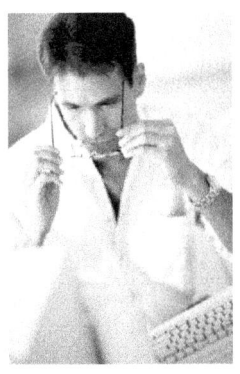

Chapter 12 Electronic Health Records (EHR)

Increasingly, healthcare providers are incorporating computer-generated or electronic health records. There are pros and cons to this method of charting.

Costs

There is governmental money available to help hospitals, doctors and other healthcare professionals to develop and implement electronic health records. It is not nearly enough. Start-up costs for transition to electronic medical records represent a large financial burden for facilities and practices.

Facilities that do not make meaningful efforts to adopt electronic health records by 2015 will be fined. Health care is an information business. Without having all the information available to everyone who needs it at the point of care, care cannot be either cost-effective or high quality. The enormous amount of data that are collected about a person's health can be stored and organized in a more efficient method than our current paper system permits.

Advantages

Placement of bar codes on medical record forms permits a handwritten form to be scanned and saved in the correct section of an electronic chart.

The electronic medical record could lead to a more efficient transfer of information from one healthcare provider to another. When using manual methods of documentation, duplication of testing and data collection can occur during care transfer from one provider to another. Cost containment and healthcare reform mandate improving efficiency in the management of healthcare data.

An electronic record may be simultaneously viewed by more than one person. The electronic medical record can be accessed by authorized people located at a remote site. For example, the physician managing the care of a nursing home resident or hospital patient can access laboratory results, orders, and medical and nursing documentation in order to make clinical decisions.

Computerized documentation supports economical use of the data entry process by reducing or eliminating redundant charting. A one-time entry of a piece of information into the program can be sent to all of the appropriate places. Copying of medical records prior to transferring a patient to a different facility can be eliminated under the electronic health record model. This system would permit the receiving facility's providers to be able to access the information gathered at the sending facility.

Hospital bedside monitors, laboratory equipment, and other devices provide data which may be electronically incorporated into the patient's medical record. The ability to review records of prior hospitalizations permits the healthcare team to obtain data about prior medical problems. There is 20-50% waste in any healthcare system. EHRs help to remove some of that waste.

Pen and paper medical records are plagued by illegible handwriting along with non-standardized and dangerous abbreviations, which can lead to medical errors. Electronic records are legible and are programmed to use only approved terminology and abbreviations.

Electronic medical records may be supplemented with resources, such as information about medications, which is useful when prescribing drugs. Systems that include data from laboratory systems can incorporate clinical prompts, for example, which may warn against prescribing a specific medication in the presence of declining kidney or liver function.

Programs can be designed to include unit-specific and disease-specific standards of care and practice. The effect of these programs is to remind the provider of the essential elements that must be documented, through the use of clinical flags.

Access to a medical record may be electronically limited. For example, a medical assistant may be permitted to only record symptoms but not review orders, laboratory results, or write nursing notes. In contrast, a paper medical record may be viewed by anyone.

Each entry in the electronic medical record carries a time and date stamp, as well as the identity of the user.
Tampering with the medical record is much more difficult to do with an electronic system. Software typically permits the healthcare professional to correct errors in typing and phrasing immediately after the error is made. Software programs contain a feature that makes the entry unalterable after a certain time or event.

With sufficient safeguards in place, an electronic record is more reliable and less likely to be lost.

One of the most obvious benefits is the creation of legible records. Computer printed records are completely legible, therefore eliminating the confusion caused by guessing at the meaning of handwritten words.

The identities of the healthcare providers are easy to determine, as each entry is followed by either initials or a full name and status MD, RN, LPN and so on). If the entry is followed by initials, somewhere else in the document the person's full name will appear.

Confidentiality Concerns

Computerized medical records pose new challenges to the healthcare provider's ethical and legal obligation to safeguard confidential information and comply with the provisions of the HIPAA.

Dedicated hackers may breach the security of electronic health records, gaining access to potentially embarrassing details about an individual.

Cautions

There are many vendors who use different platforms, with only minimal efforts at standardization. A healthcare complex may contain different types of electronic health records which are incompatible and cannot share information with each other, such as the emergency department, labor and delivery and the radiology department. The lack of standardization means that it is very difficult to share information from one practice setting to another (such as one physician office to another) or from the physician office to the acute care setting.

Failure to authenticate a medical record may permit alterations of data after the entry should have become permanent. Authentication finishes a record entry, making it permanent. For example, a nurse who fails to authenticate nursing notes until the end of an eight hour shift may make changes after an event has occurred.

Most EHR software systems have the ability to "auto-populate" data fields. In this situation, a key data element, such as an allergy to penicillin, need only be entered into the record once. It will be automatically entered into every other area of the record which requires allergy information. When the wrong information is entered into one of these key fields, that error will be auto-populated throughout the record and may cause medical errors.

Computer systems may become unavailable due to unexpected crashes or routine downtime. Medical information becomes inaccessible during these times, creating potential for medical errors. All ambulatory practices which have converted to EHR need to have tested protocols which allow all practitioners to continue documenting smoothly during those times when the EHR system is "down".

Physician and nursing resistance to the use of computers is a factor that complicates the introduction of computers to a healthcare setting. Partial use of the computer and partial use of handwritten entries can create a confusing record.

The adage "garbage in, garbage out" applies to the computer medical record just as it does to other aspects of computer programming. Healthcare personnel must guard against the temptation to deify the computer. Meaningless documentation can also be generated when templates are used without modification or individualization. There are dangers in using templates, or copying and pasting information into an EHR system. There are dangers in providers sharing logins. There are dangers in providers modifying or deleting electronic entries after the fact of treatment. There are dangers in a hospital having several EHR systems that do not communicate with each other. Data can be corrupted or lost.

In some systems, physicians who do not detect any changes in the patient's condition from the previous visit may automatically insert the documentation from the previous visit. This feature saves time but can be a trap for if the physician fails to conduct the assessment.

Systems can be cumbersome to use. Staff can adopt dangerous work arounds which subvert the safety systems. For example, a nurse in Wisconsin bypassed the safety features of bar scanning medical compliance software and killed a 16 year old pregnant mother who received an infusion that was intended for the epidural route but instead got the medication into her peripheral IV. The nurse did not place an identification band on the patient, which was required to use the bar coding system to match the drugs with the selected drug. She failed to use the bar coding system. The department nurses had collectively practiced deviating from the protocols. The department training on the software was suboptimal. The technology was recently implemented and not fully functional. The protocols were perceived as not urgent in contrast to the normal patient demands in the labor and delivery unit.

Key Documentation Points
1. Position yourself when you chart in the presence of the patient to face the patient or at least to have the opportunity to maintain eye contact. Patients can feel depersonalized when they see a staff member absorbed in the computer.
2. Take care to ensure you are charting in the correct records.
3. Beware of the tendency to fall into a pattern of rote charting. Each click has meaning and should convey accurate information.

4. Do not share your password and login information with anyone. One nurse I counseled was reported to the board of nursing for logging onto the computer using another nurse's password – for six months. This means that all of the medical chart entries he created were under the name of another person.
5. Be very careful if you copy and paste information from one entry to the next. Make sure it is current and accurate.
6. Do not give into the temptation to work around the safety features of the software.

Computer Prescriber Order Entry (CPOE)

Orders written by computers have the advantage of being legible. Decision software in the program can prevent accepting an order that is incorrect. When the ordering software is integrated with the laboratory software, it can check current liver and kidney test results to verify that a medication toxic to the kidneys and liver can be safely given. Let's consider two examples of why computer physician order entry is so important.

Case Example

In a California case, the fifty-five year-old plaintiff underwent surgery to repair a torn tendon. The podiatrist performed the procedure at a hospital and planned to have the patient go to a subacute rehabilitation center. He wrote an order for Morphine 50 mg IM for postoperative pain at the time of her discharge. The drug was not given before she left the hospital. When the patient arrived at the subacute facility and the staff processed the order, the pharmacy told the nurses that the Morphine order was unusually high. The facility's administration authorized the nurse to proceed with the morphine injection without the approval of the patient's attending physician. (The podiatrist did not have privileges at the subacute facility.)

The staff searched the facility to obtain all of the Morphine which was available and injected 30 mg at 5:30 PM. The next morning the patient was found unresponsive due to an overdose of Morphine, which caused a heart attack, renal failure and anoxic brain injury. The plaintiff requires 24-hour care.

The plaintiff alleged negligence by the official attending physician and the physician covering for the official attending physician in that there was a failure to act as the attending physician and negligence in signing the Morphine order after the fact. Those physicians settled prior to trial. The plaintiff maintained that the facility's policies required medication orders to be approved by the attending physician, but the staff did not obtain his approval for the Morphine order. The plaintiff additionally maintained that no chart entries were made at the time of the Morphine administration and that the nurses involved were required to create documents after she was sent to the emergency room. The plaintiff also claimed there was a lack of monitoring of the plaintiff.

The podiatrist claimed he intended the order to be for Demerol and mistakenly wrote Morphine and admitted liability, but maintained that the order was actually only a recommendation, as he did not have privileges at the facility where it was administered. The nurse who administered the injection admitted he knew at the time that the dose was too high, but did not increase monitoring or make any charge notes before leaving the facility that day because he was too busy. The facility claimed the administration of Morphine was proper because it was performed pursuant to a physician's order.

The jury awarded $3,189,005 in damages. The jury also supported finding punitive damages against the facility. The case settled for a confidential amount before the punitive damages phase of the trial. [89]

Comment: Had the podiatrist entered the order into a computer, the safety alerts in the software should have flagged this order.

Case Example

This is an example from a case that involved a 17-year-old girl who was being treated for bone cancer. She was on this regimen of methotrexate and leucovorin.

The oncologist hand calculated the dose for each of the 12 treatments. There were no order sets. There were no protocols. In every order, there were scratch outs and number changes. The methotrexate was supposed to be given for 4 hours and then leucovorin was the rescue drug to be given to help neutralize the effects of the methotrexate. It was supposed to be started 16 hours after the completion of the dose and to be given every 3 hours for eight doses. Note that the dose of the leucovorin was 240 mg.

On the 12th treatment, the doctor changed the order and instead of giving leucovorin 240 mg, he ordered 38 mg. He also changed the rest of the order so it was to begin at 18 hours after the methotrexate dose and to be given every 6 hours. He didn't do this intentionally. The patient received her dose of methotrexate; it ran for 5 1/2 hours instead of the 4 hours that was ordered.

PATIENT CARE DOCUMENTATION RECORD

DATE / TIME	FOCUS / NURSING DIAGNOSIS	PATIENT CARE NOTES D - Data • A - Action • R - Response
1500	admissions	D) Pt admitted to 1228, – ambulatory. Pt c̄ 90 of pain. ___ signature
2300	chemotherapy	A) IV started into (L) lower arm. Excellent blood return. IV fluids started. Chemo started c̄ Mtx. @ 250. CSh
0430	chemo complete	Chemo complete. D5 ½ NS 2amp. Pacu?? @ 125. ___ CSh

Regional Medical Center

Phoenix, AZ

NURSING UNIT	ROOM - BED

CHEMOTHERAPY ORDER SHEET

SECTION 1: PATIENT CLINICAL INFORMATION (Complete A-E):

A. DIAGNOSIS _Osteosarcoma_

B. HEIGHT _64_ INCHES _____ CM   C. WEIGHT _____ LBS _83.5_ KG

D. BODY SURFACE AREA (M²) _1.9 m²_

E. PROTOCOL OR REFERENCE FOR REGIMEN _H.D. MTX_
(IF APPLICABLE)

SECTION 2: CHEMOTHERAPY MEDICATIONS (GENERIC NAME ONLY - NO ABBREVIATIONS)

	MEDICATION	DOSAGE mg/M² or mg/Kg	ROUTE	DOSE TO BE GIVEN	SOLUTION/VOLUME/ ADD'L INGREDIENTS	FREQUENCY/ DURATION
C H E M O T H E R A P Y	Methotrexate	12 g/m² (grams)	IV	20 gm	(Max Dose)	Over 4° x1
	Leucovorin	20 ug/m²	IV	240 mg		Begin 16° p completion of MTX @ 3° x 8 doses

176

CHEMOTHERAPY ORDER SHEET

SECTION 1: PATIENT CLINICAL INFORMATION (Complete A-E):

A. DIAGNOSIS _Osteosarcoma_

B. HEIGHT _____ INCHES _____ CM   C. WEIGHT _____ LBS _____ KG

D. BODY SURFACE AREA (M²) _____ 1.9 m²

E. PROTOCOL OR REFERENCE FOR REGIMEN _____
   (IF APPLICABLE)

SECTION 2: CHEMOTHERAPY MEDICATIONS (GENERIC NAME ONLY - NO ABBREVIATIONS)

	MEDICATION	DOSAGE mg/M² or mg/kg	ROUTE	DOSE TO BE GIVEN	SOLUTION/VOLUME/ ADD'L INGREDIENTS	FREQUENCY/ DURATION
C	Methotrexate	10g/m²	IV	20gm	in 1L D5W	over 40
H	Leucovorin	20mg/m²	IV	38mg	⟶	q 6° x Please
E						beginning 180
M						after MTX
O						completed
T						
H						
E						
R						
A						
P						
Y						

The mother was at the bedside; she had been at the bedside of her daughter for every one of these treatments and she knew that the leucovorin needed to be started sooner and to be given more frequently. She questioned the nurse. The nurse said, "It's in the middle of the night, I can't wake up a doctor to question this. You'll have to wait until the morning."

By the morning, it was too late. The girl developed toxic epidermal necrolysis, which meant that all of her skin was sloughed off and she died from an overwhelming infection. This case settled out of court. Had the physician been able to use CPOE, the protocol would have been selected from a standard order set, and he would not have had to hand calculate every order.

There are some drawbacks to CPOE. Incomplete or inaccurate order sets, hurdles to adoption and lack of testing can turn a CPOE system that is supposed to improve patient safety into one that puts patients at risk of being injured. CPOE is not faster or easier for providers than written or verbal orders. Setting up too many alerts can make CPOE difficult for providers to navigate. They start to tune them out and click through them without paying attention.

It is possible to determine who accesses an EHR and what screens this person reviewed. Metadata is data about data. It indicates how and when a computer or application was used and by which person. The query audit trail or medical record review inquiry details who looked at the medical record, when and for how long and whether the hard copy of the medical record left the medical records department. The audit trail includes the additions, deletions, and edits for the time frame at issue. It identifies which people documented when.

Case Example
A patient began bleeding after surgery. Her physician claimed the nurses did not tell her about the dropping hemoglobin and hematocrit. The metadata, however, showed the physician opened up the patient's lab results and reviewed them. The jury found the physician negligent.

Chapter 13 Summary

This book focuses on the role of the medical record and litigation and why people sue. You have learned some of the factors that contribute to errors. Here are some conclusions: if you're not sure ask a more experienced person; always seek some assistance if you're not clear. Be a patient advocate; people count on you to ask those questions. Chart as completely as you can. Remember the chart's going to be scrutinized if there is a bad outcome and the patient seeks a plaintiff attorney.

Don't omit details of care or treatment that you provided, particularly the important aspects of care that relate to why the patient received care in your area. Don't omit any details of an incident. Don't do finger pointing or blame others; chart just the objective details, what was done, and who was contacted.

Remember that although computer prescriber order entry provides benefits it also has some draw backs. Use your critical thinking to evaluate what you see on the screen in front of you. Electronic prescriptions which are created by the physician, nurse practitioner, or physician's assistant have the advantage of being legible, backed by standards and connections to other aspects of the medical record. They bring their own advantages and disadvantages, they offer some important patient safety safeguards. So if you are concerned about the struggles and the traumas associated with implementing computer physician order entry, remember the hazards of handwritten orders. As you transition into that role, keep in mind that this a much safer system for providing orders. We have all incorporated computers into our lives whether they are phones, answering machines, or charts and we tend to rely on them. But remember somebody could have sat down and ordered this on the wrong patient, could have been thinking about somebody else.

As you answer calls from patients, it is always important to use your critical thinking and ask questions. Keep the physician informed of significant changes in the patient's condition and don't hesitate to use the chain of command until you're satisfied that you've gotten an answer.

SBAR: Creating Clear Communication

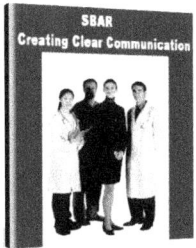

Patricia W. Iyer

52 pages, e-book (download)

Attention Healthcare Providers: If you have been wanting to learn how SBAR helps improve communication and saves patient lives, you must read this ebook!

Finally! An easy to understand guide that will make communicating with SBAR easy.

Dear Fellow Healthcare Provider,

- Are you frustrated by medical errors?
- Do you see patients being injured because of miscommunication?
- Do you long for a method of easily communicating the important information when you turn care over to another provider?
- Are you searching for ways to improve team work?
- Do you want to reduce your risk of being sued for malpractice?

There are lots of books on medical errors but few on a simple technique that saves lives. For the last 25 years of working with attorneys, I have heard case after case of patients being injured by miscommunication. So I decided to write a book called *SBAR: Creating Clear Communication*. It is like no other book ever written. And you can't buy it at Amazon or Barnes and Noble.

Here's what you'll learn after reading *SBAR: Creating Clear Communication*:

- What SBAR is different from SOAP charting

- How you can use SBAR to reduce medical errors

- Why SBAR promotes clear communication between providers

- How SBAR improves your listening skills

- How SBAR will simplify your hand-offs

- Why SBAR will help you avoid being sued

- How you can flawlessly implement SBAR

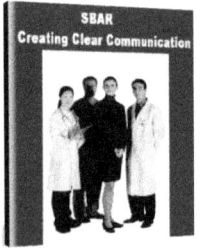

But that's not all! You will also receive:

- Answers to frequently asked questions

- A list of essential resources

- Sample forms

- Tips for training others in SBAR

- Optional 20 nursing contact hours (for a nominal additional cost of $20.00)*

Here is what your colleagues had to say about *SBAR: Creating Clear Communication*:

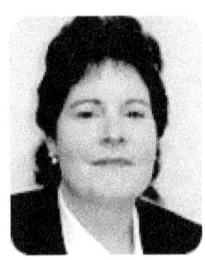

"What an outstanding resource this is! It is really excellent! We have been using the SBAR technique since January 2009 and have found it to be very 'user friendly', especially with newer staff. The short time needed to use the SBAR technique will pay off in the end by creating a standard for which all communication is based. I find that today's newer staff members need an easy, reliable, and standardized procedure like this." — *Christina Turner RN, Administrative Resource Coordinator, Chambersburg Hospital, PA*

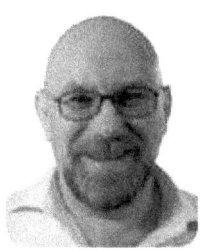

"Very interesting and well done. On the front lines of patient care we need tools that make sense. SBAR is simply a better way of communicating."
— *Larry Cohen MD FCCP FCCM*
Associate Professor of Anesthesiology, Medicine & Surgery, State University of New York @ Buffalo
Associate Director, Critical Care, Roswell Park Cancer Institute

The only way to purchase this 52-page ebook is on our website. And in just 90 seconds, you can download it to your computer right now. So as soon as you place your order, you will have instant access to it. No waiting in the mail for the book to show up.

I want you to be happy with your purchase. If you are not satisfied that my book I want you to keep the book and I will refund the money. **This is my 100% guarantee:** That's how much confidence I have in knowing you'll love the book.

Order with credit card or Paypal through our secure webstore at www.legalnursebusiness.com

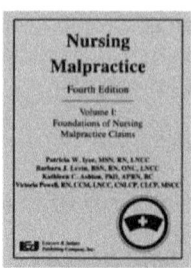

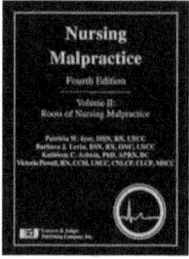

Nursing Malpractice, Fourth Edition
Edited by Patricia Iyer, MSN, RN, LNCC
Barbara Levin, BSN, RN, ONC, LNCC,
Kathleen Ashton, PhD, APRN, BC,
Victoria Powell, RN, CCM, LNCC,
CNLCP, CLCP, MSCC, CEASII

2 volumes, casebound, 2011, Lawyers
and Judges

Volume I (Beige), 736 pages

Volume II (Blue), 960 pages

Order at legalnursebusiness.com

Patricia Iyer and her coeditors Barbara Levin, Kathleen Ashton, and Victoria Powell, are proud (and relieved) to announce the new edition of *Nursing Malpractice*. An outstanding reference for the attorney, legal nurse consultant, insurance claim adjuster, healthcare risk manager, or healthcare facility leader involved in a nursing malpractice claim, the fourth edition of *Nursing Malpractice* brings you a wealth of information and resources for your case. This extensively revised and updated edition of a classic covers the spectrum of the nursing process. Packed with tips and techniques this volume reveals a comprehensive overview of nursing responsibilities.

Untangling Charlotte's Web: A Case Study

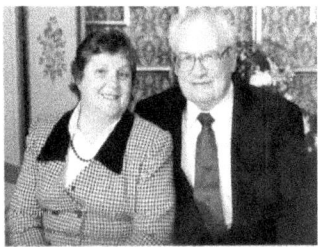 One woman's healthcare journey resulted in profound changes both within a hospital system and within the United States. Her complications have affected patients throughout the country - her case influenced the development of the Joint Commission National Patient Safety Goal regarding reporting critical lab results. The presenters have carried Charlotte's message to nurses and physicians both nationally and internationally.

This case study described how a series of errors culminated in her cardiac arrest. The program uses slides, video clips and photos to tell the story of how nursing, laboratory and physicians contributed to her arrest and brain damage.

Format: DVD of a gripping 80 minute presentation in front of a nursing audience. This program is perfect for an educational program for staff.

"Every day tens if not hundreds of thousands of errors occur in the healthcare system," according to the Institute of Medicine, and "some cause disastrous effects." Errors are costly to patients, hospitals and insurance companies. A collaborative approach towards patient safety involves all members of the healthcare team. Communication issues are the leading contributing factors resulting in patient injury.

This program tells the story of how one patient, Charlotte, was profoundly affected by miscommunication. There are a multitude of facets which will be addressed and include inexperience, generational, and communication styles. Specific guidance on the use of communication to avoid unexpected events will be provided. This program will utilize a case study approach. The participant will have an opportunity to see the application of the Swiss Cheese model as the presenters detail the breakdown in communication which resulted in a sentinel event and cardiac arrest. This extraordinary program will affect every attendee. Photos and videos will be shared detailing this unexpected and near fatal event.

Topics discussed in this program include SBAR communication, workplace bullying, generational values, and patient advocacy. The audience will learn what an institution did to incorporate new policies and procedures and education to safeguard lives.

Order at legalnursebusiness.com

Price: $97

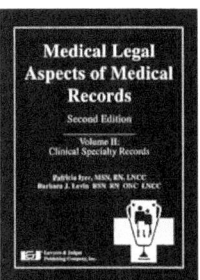

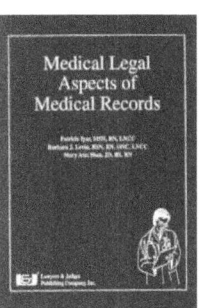

Medical Legal Aspects of Medical Records

Patricia Iyer RN, MSN, LNCC, Barbara Levin BSN RN LNCC, Mary Ann Shea RN JD

2010, 8.5" x 11", casebound

**Volume I (Blue), 416 pages
Volume II (Green), 672 pages**

Order at:
www.legalnursebusiness.com

A critical reference for understanding medical records.

This comprehensive book sheds light on the complex world of medical records. Although the book originally was intended to focus just on medical records, each author took advantage of the opportunity to provide a wider glimpse into the subject matter. Thus, the reader will come away from this book gaining broader knowledge about healthcare delivery, which will assist in analyzing medical records and details. The text is intended to benefit attorneys, paralegals, legal nurse consultants, risk managers, and anyone else with a keen appreciation of the nuances of medical records.

End notes

[1] Laska, L. (Ed.) "Man dies after sitting in family physician's exam room for forty minutes after complaining of chest pain", *Medical Malpractice Verdicts, Settlements, and Experts*, October 2011, page 18.

[2] "Failure to properly evaluate man suffering from throat pain with abnormal EKG", *Medical Malpractice Verdicts, Settlements and Experts*, March 2010, page 11.

[3] Croke, E. "Nurses, negligence, and malpractice", *American Journal of Nursing*, September 2003, 103 (9), pages 54-63.

[4] *Telehealth Nursing Practice Administration and Practice Standards*, American Academy of Ambulatory Care Nursing, 2007, Pitman, NJ.

[5] *The Role of the Registered Nurse in Ambulatory Care Position Statement*, American Academy of Ambulatory Care Nursing, December 2010.

[6] Laska, L. (Ed.) "Failure to perform EKG and refer for cardiac evaluation", *Medical Malpractice Verdicts, Settlements and Experts*, January 2010, page 22.

[7] Ambulatory Care National Patient Safety Goals, The Joint Commission Accreditation of Ambulatory Care, www.jointcommission.org.

[8] ECRI, Top 10 Technology Hazards for 2012, www.ecri.org/2012_Top_10_hazards.

[9] Iyer, P. "Roots of Patient Injury", in Iyer, P., Levin, B., Ashton, K. and Powell, V. (Editors), *Nursing Malpractice*, Fourth Edition, Lawyers and Judges Publishing Company, 2011. Available through www.legalnursebusiness.com.

[10] Laska, L. (Ed), "Failure to timely diagnose lung cancer", *Medical Malpractice Verdicts, Settlements and Experts*, December 2007, pages 7-8.

[11] Barrett, J, Gifford, C., Morey, J, Risser, D., and Salisbury, M., "Enhancing patient safety through teamwork training", *Journal of Healthcare Risk Management*, Fall 2001, pages 57-65.

[12] Iyer, P, and Camp, N. *Nursing Documentation*, Fourth Edition, Med League, Flemington, NJ, 2004, available through www.legalnursebusiness.com.

[13] Laska, L. (Ed), "Bladder ruptures following prostate surgery", *Medical Malpractice Verdicts, Settlements and Experts*, January 2008, page 51.

[14] American Nurses Association, *Scope and Standards of Nursing Practice*, Washington, DC: The Author, page 38, 2004.

[15] Laska, L. (Ed.) "Man claims he wasn't properly monitored during procedure to place prosthetic lens", *Medical Malpractice Verdicts, Settlements, and Experts*, September 2011, page 3.

[16] Laska, L. (Ed.), "Man found dead from narcotic overdose two days after visit to clinic", *Medical Malpractice Verdicts, Settlements, and Experts*, December 2011, page 16.

[17] Jones, J. "Chain of command: a risk management perspective", *Compass*, March 2004, http://www.mcneary.com/pdf/consortium_newsletters/Vol2No2Compas s.pdf, accessed March 9, 2008.

[18] Reising, D. and Allen, P. "Protecting yourself from malpractice claims", *American Nurse Today*, February 2007, page 39.

[19] Laska, L. (Ed), "Failure to contact physician when man complains of severe back pain while hospitalized for regulation of blood coagulation following aortic valve graft surgery", *Medical Malpractice Verdicts, Settlements, and Experts*, January 2006. Page 17.

[20] Lisa Black, "Original research: tragedy into policy" *American Journal of Nursing*, June 2011, Vol 111, No. 6.

[21] From a blog post written by Patricia Iyer for www.avoidmedicalerrors.com.

[22] http://www.jointcommission.org/SentinelEvents/SentinelEventAlert/sea _24.htm

23

http://www.jointcommission.org/SentinelEvents/SentinelEventAlert/sea_24.htm

[24] http://www.projo.com/news/content/WRONG_Site_11-27-07_PB818Q7_v12.2704b40.html

[25] McCorkle, D. and Pietro, J., "Perioperative nursing malpractice issues", in Iyer, P. , Levin, B., Ashton, K. and Powell, V. (Eds), *Nursing Malpractice*, Fourth Edition, Lawyers and Judges Publishing Company, 2011.

[26] ECRI, Operating Room Risk Management Surgery, 23, November 2003, pages 1-15.

27

http://www.jointcommission.org/SentinelEvents/SentinelEventAlert/sea_7.htm

28

http://www.jointcommission.org/SentinelEvents/SentinelEventAlert/sea_14.htm

[29] Laska, L. (Ed). "Failure to conduct ordered checks and keep psychiatric patient under proper observation", *Medical Malpractice Verdicts, Settlements, and Experts*, January 2008, page 43.

[30] Laska, L. (Ed.) "Failure to properly monitor woman with diagnosis of delirium", *Medical Malpractice Verdicts, Settlements, and Experts*, July 2007, page 20.

[31] "Risk management issues in assessing suicidal and homicidal patients", *Journal of Healthcare Risk Management*, Vol. 27, No. 3, 2008, page 42.

[32] See www.ismp.org/Tools/highalertmedications.pdf

[33] Moore, T, Cohen, M. and Furberg, C. "Serious adverse drug events reported to the Food and Drug Administration, 1998-2005", *Archives of Internal Medicine*, 167, No. 16, September 10, 2007, pages 1752-1759.

[34] Laska, L. (Ed.) "Young woman given massive overdose of Acetylcystine for Tylenol overdose", *Medical Malpractice Verdicts, Settlements, and Experts*, November 2011, pages 9-10.

[35] Laska, L. (Ed,) "Woman claims loss of consciousness after influenza vaccination caused auto crash", *Malpractice Verdicts, Settlements, and Experts*, January 2010, page 10.

[36] Laska, L. (Ed.)"Failure to provide pneumococcal vaccine for woman without spleen", *Medical Malpractice Verdicts, Settlements and Experts*, January 2010, page 20.

[37] www.ismp.org/msarticles/council.htm

[38] O'Donnell, J., Cohen, I.L. and Iyer, P. "Medication Errors and Adverse Drug Reactions In Hospitals, From A Medico-Legal Perspective", in O'Donnell, J. (Editor), *Drug Injury: Liability, Analysis, And Prevention*, Second Edition, Tucson, AZ: Lawyers and Judges Publishing Company, 2005. Available through www.medleague.com.

[39] Laska, L. (Ed.) Failure to diagnose appendicitis in young child blamed for death", *Medical Malpractice verdicts, Settlements and Experts*, January 2010, page 32.

[40] American Nurses Association. *Implementing Nursing's Report Card: A Study of RN Staffing, Length of Stay and Patient Outcomes*. Washington DC, The Author, 1997.

[41] Esparaza, S., Zoller, J, White, A. and Highfield, M. "Nurse staffing and skill mix patterns: are there differences in outcomes?" *Journal of Healthcare Risk Management*, Vol. 31, No. 3, pages 14-21.

[42] Kovner, C. and Gergen, P. "Nurse staffing levels and adverse events following surgery in U.S. hospitals." *Image-The Journal of Nursing Scholarship*. 30 (4), 1998. Page 315.

[43] Needleman, J., Mattke, S. et al, *Nurse Staffing Levels and Patient Outcomes in Hospitals. Final Report for Health Resources and Services Administration*, Contract No. 230-99-0021, 2001. Harvard School of Public Health, Boston, MA, as quoted in "Hospital Nurse Staffing and Quality of Care," www.ahrq.gov. March 2004.

[44] Aiken, L., Sloane, D. Lake, E., et al "Hospital nurse staffing and patient mortality" *JAMA*, 288 (16): October 23/30, 2002, pages 1987-1993.

[45] Laska, L. (Ed.) "Failure to diagnose Fournier's Gangrene of groin, buttocks, and abdomen despite repeated visits to emergency room and clinic", *Medical Malpractice Verdicts, Settlements, and Experts*, January 2010, page 7.

[46] Laska, L. (Ed), "Hypoxic brain damage to infant", *Medical Malpractice Verdicts, Settlements, and Experts*, March 2003, page 34.

[47] Rosenstein, A. and O' Daniel, M. "Disruptive behavior and clinical outcomes: perceptions of nurses and physicians", *AJN*, 105: 1, January 2005, pages 54-63.

[48] Mason, D. "Safe practices and quality health care", presentation at 3rd Annual Patient Safety Conference: University of Pennsylvania, December 1, 2005.

[49] DuBose, J. and Donahue, T. "Taking the pain out of patient handling", *American Nurse Today*, December 2006, pages 37-42.

[50] Laska, L. (Ed.) "Woman suffers fractured ankle when chair with rollers rolls out from under her when she is being prepared for laser surgery", *Medical Malpractice Verdicts, Settlements and Experts*, September 2011, page 25.

[51] Kane, R., Burns, E. and Goodwin, J., "Minimal trauma fractures in older nursing home residents: the interaction of functional status, trauma, and site of fracture", *The American Geriatrics Society*, 43, 1995, pages 156-159.

[52] Martin-Hunyadi, C., "Clinical and prognostic aspects of spontaneous fractures in long term care units: a thirty-month prospective study", *Revue de Medecine Interne*, 21 (9), September 2000.

[53] Laska, L. (Ed), "Colonoscopy patient falls from bed before procedure starts", *Medical Malpractice Verdicts, Settlements, and Experts*, January 2006, page 14.

[54] Pullen, R. "Screening for abuse and neglect", *Nursing 2007*, February 2007, page 69.

[55] Burgess, A., Brown, K, Bell, K, Ledray, L, and Poarch, J., "Sexual abuse of older adults", *American Journal of Nursing*, October 2005, page 66.

[56] Capezuti, E. and Swedlow, D., "Sexual abuse in nursing homes", *Elder's Advisor*, Fall 2000, page 51.

[57] Foa, E. and Rothbau, B, *Treating the Trauma of Rape*, New York, The Guilford Press, 1998.

[58] Fields, R. "Severe stress and the elderly: Are older adults at increased risk for posttraumatic stress disorder?" In P. Ruskin and J. Talbott, (Eds), *Aging and Posttraumatic Stress Disorder*, Washington, DC American Psychiatric Press, 1996.

[59] See also Rom-Rymer, B, "Demonstrating trauma- effects of sexual abuse on the elderly", in Krisztal, R. *Nursing Home Litigation: Pretrial Practice and Trials*, Second Edition, Lawyers and Judges, 2003. Available at www.medleague.com.

[60] Laska, L. (Ed), "Elderly woman raped at nursing home and also subjected to multiple non-sexual assaults", *Medical Malpractice Verdicts, Settlements, and Experts*, August 2003, page 36.

[61] Laska, L. (Ed), "Sexual assault on woman in ICU of Army Hospital", *Medical Malpractice Verdicts, Settlements, and Experts*, April 2006, pages 21-22.

[62] McCorkle, D. and Pietro, J. "Perioperative nursing malpractice issues" in Iyer, P., Levin, B., Ashton, K. and Powell, V. (Eds). *Nursing Malpractice*, Fourth Edition, Lawyers and Judges Publishing Company, 2011. Available at www.legalnursebusiness.com.

[63] Laska, L. (Ed.), "Woman claims laparotomy pad left after cesarean section caused ulcerative colitis", *Medical Malpractice Verdicts, Settlements, and Experts*, December 2011, page 25.

[64]
http://www.jointcommission.org/SentinelEvents/SentinelEventAlert/sea_25.htm

[65] Ashton, K. and Beerman, J. "Critical Care Malpractice Issues" in Iyer, P., Levin, B., Ashton, K. and Powell, V. (Eds), *Nursing Malpractice*, Fourth Edition, Lawyers and Judges Publishing Company, 2011, available at www.legalnursebusiness.com.

66
http://www.jointcommission.org/SentinelEvents/SentinelEventAlert/sea_25.htm

[67] Laska, L. (Ed.), "Man dies from cardiac arrest in ICU when monitor alarms not hear and faulty wiring prevents alert on central monitors", *Medical Malpractice Verdicts, Settlements and Experts,* October 2011, page 16.

[68] Feutz-Harter, S. *Legal and Ethical Standards for Nurses,* PESI, 2006.

[69] Laska, L. (Ed.) "Hospital settles for $4.9 million after man suffers brain damage from respiratory distress while being treated for epiglottitis", *Medical Malpractice Verdicts, Settlements, and Experts,* November 2011, page 15.

[70] Aiken, T. and Catalano, J. *Legal, Ethical, and Political Issues in Nursing,* FA Davis, Philadelphia, 1994.

[71] Greene, P. "The defense attorney's perspective" in Iyer, P., Levin. B., Ashton, K. and Powell, V. *Nursing Malpractice,* Fourth Edition, Lawyers and Judge Publishing Company, 2011. Available at www.medleague.com.

[72] Laska, L. (Ed.) "Woman found in another patient's room with blood on face and assault-like injuries following abdominal surgery", *Medical Malpractice Verdicts, Settlements, and Experts,* January 2010, page 19.

[73] Laska, L. (Ed.) "Failure to replace IV when cap becomes dislodged blamed for development of MRSA and death", *Medical Malpractice Verdicts, Settlements, and Experts,* December 2011, page 13.

[74] Capezuti, E. and Swedlow, D. "Sexual abuse in nursing homes", *Elder's Advisor,* Fall, 2000, page 51.

[75] Laska, L. (Ed), "Home health company's employee fails to stay with physically and mentally handicapped woman during dialysis catheter pulled from chest", *Medical Malpractice Verdicts, Settlements, and Experts,* April 2006, pages 22-23.

[76] Austin, S. "Seven legal tips for safe nursing practice", *Nursing 2008,* March 2008, page 35.

[77] Reising, D. and Allen, P., "Protecting yourself from malpractice claims", *American Nurse Today,* February 2007, page 39.

[78] Laska, L. (Ed.) "Failure to notice and treat leg laceration", *Medical Malpractice Verdicts, Settlements, and Experts*, April 2006, page 34.

[79] Hughes, R and Stone, P, "The perils of shift work", *American Journal of Nursing*, 104 (9), September 2004, pages 60-63.

[80] Labyak, S. et al "Effects of shift work on sleep and menstrual function in nurses," *Health Care Women Int*: 23, 6-7, 2002, pages 703-714.

[81] Baxter, L. and Seltzer, M. "Health care professional impairment", *Legal Medicine*, Sixth Edition, Mosby, St. Louis, 2004.

[82] Carruth, A. and Booth, D. "Disciplinary actions against nurses: Who is at risk?" *Journal of Nursing Law*, 6 (3), p. 55, November 1999.

[83] Aiken, T. and Catalano, J. *Legal, Ethical, and Political Issues in Nursing*, FA Davis Company, Philadelphia, 1994.

[84] Clifford, R., Grogan, A., and Leverock, M., "Significance of healthcare fraud in nursing", in Iyer, P., Levin, B., Ashton, K. and Powell, V. (Editors), *Nursing Malpractice*, Fourth Edition, Lawyers and Judges Publishing Company, 2011. Available at www.legalnursebusiness.com.

[85] Murray, J. "Before blowing the whistle, learn to protect yourself", *American Nurse Today*, March 2007, page 40.

[86] *Telehealth Nursing Practice Administration and Practice Standards*, Standard V, American Academy of Ambulatory Care Nursing, 2007, Pitman, NJ. 38. "$200K for HIV Test Disclosure", *New Jersey Law Journal*, October 17, 2005, page 9.

[88] Laska, L. (Ed.) "Medical office sent billing statements to attorney which showed patient's HIV positive status while seeking payment of outstanding balance", *Medical Malpractice Verdicts, Settlements and Experts*, January 2011, page 3.

[89] Laska, L. (Ed.) "Failure to properly check order for 50 milligrams of Morphine for woman following podiatric surgery", *Medical Malpractice Verdicts, Settlements and Experts*, January 2011, Page 12.

Consider Writing a Review

Thank you for buying this book. When you enjoy a book, it is a natural desire to tell others about it. Amazon.com provides a way to share your thoughts and I invite you to write a book review. It is easy. Here are tips:

1. After going to the link below on Amazon.com, the first thing you are asked to do is to assign a number of stars to the book you think matches your opinion of the book.

2. Create a title for the review. This can be a simple phrase, like "Awesome guide." If you are not sure what to say, look at the titles of other book reviews.

3. It is easiest to write the book in a word processor and then paste it into Amazon.com Your word processor will pick up typos before your review goes public.

4. Write the review as if you were talking to another person – you are – a person who comes to Amazon.com and is considering buying this book.

5. Include a description of what you found most helpful. Was it an idea, chapter, tip? Share that with the readers.

6. Next you may want to write who you think would most benefit from this book. Is it for beginners? Or is it more appropriate for someone with experience with this topic?

7. What if you have something negative to say about the book? You may always reach me at patriciaiyer@gmail.com to suggest changes in the book.

8. If you include negative feedback in the review, keep a positive perspective rather than attack the author.

Here are some sample phrases:

- While overall the book was good, I would change it by. . .
- I don't think this book is right for. . .
- I would improve this book by. . .

Before you hit save, read everything over one more time.

Authors and readers appreciate book reviews and they get easier to write with time. Go to this link on Amazon.com to write your review. If for any reason it does not work, search for the book title + Iyer and it will show.

Link: http://bit.ly/SafeguardAmbulatory

Thank you,

Pat Iyer

.

www.ingramcontent.com/pod-product-compliance
Lightning Source LLC
Chambersburg PA
CBHW051459170526
45166CB00001B/312

* 9 7 8 1 4 7 5 1 7 5 6 6 0 *